THE HEALING KITCHEN

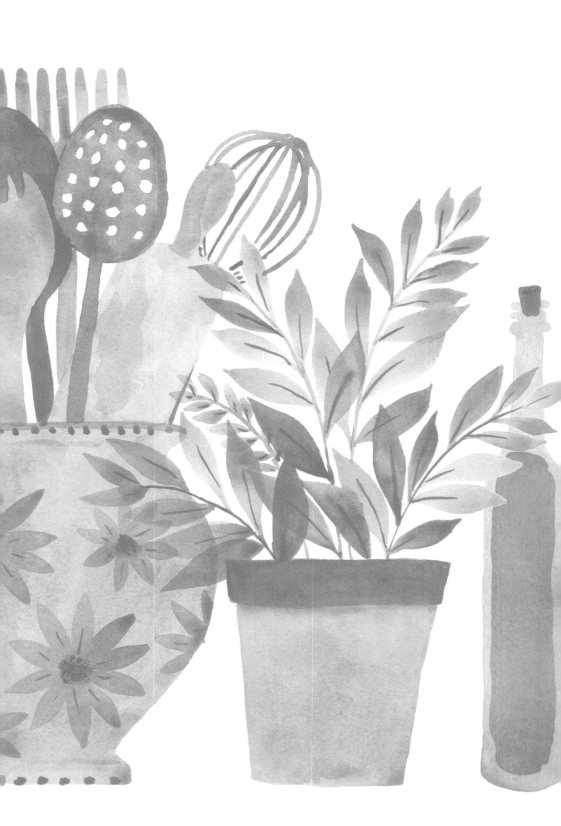

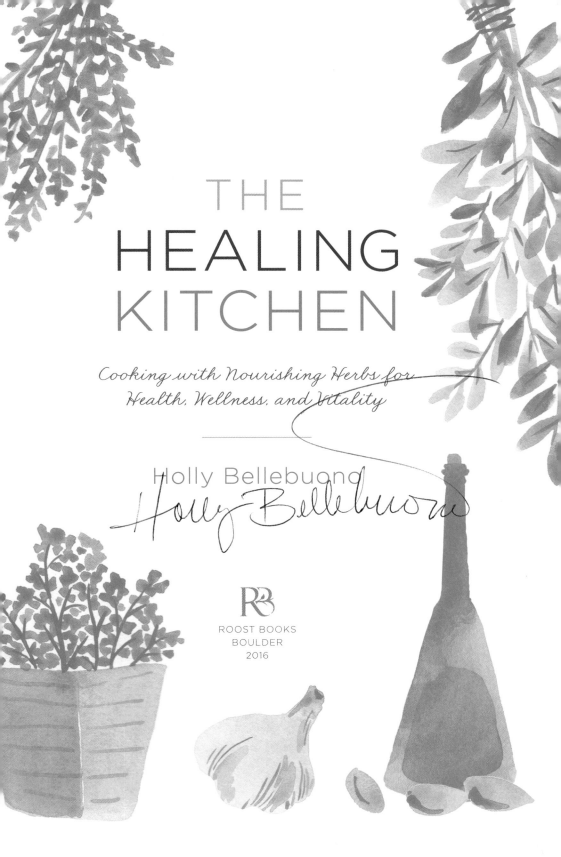

THE
HEALING
KITCHEN

Cooking with Nourishing Herbs for
Health, Wellness, and Vitality

Holly Bellebuono

Holly Bellebuono

ROOST BOOKS
BOULDER
2016

ROOST BOOKS
An imprint of Shambhala Publications, Inc.
4720 Walnut Street
Boulder, Colorado 80301
roostbooks.com

The recipes herein have been created based on personal experience and the study of a vast heritage of herbal healing. They are presented here for the enjoyment of the reader and in no instance are meant to take the place of the care of a qualified health practitioner. For health matters, please seek the advice of a trusted health care practitioner.

9 8 7 6 5 4 3 2 1

First Edition
Printed in the United States of America

⊗This edition is printed on acid-free paper that meets
the American National Standards Institute Z39.48 Standard.
♻Shambhala Publications makes every effort to print on recycled paper.
For more information please visit www.shambhala.com.

Distributed in the United States by Penguin Random House LLC
and in Canada by Random House of Canada Ltd

Designed by Laura Shaw Design, Inc.

Library of Congress Cataloging-in-Publication Data

Names: Bellebuono, Holly, author.
Title: The healing kitchen: cooking with nourishing herbs for health, wellness, and vitality/Holly Bellebuono.
Description: First edition. | Boulder: Roost Books, [2016] | Includes bibliographical references and index.
Identifiers: LCCN 2015037838 | ISBN 9781611802788 (hardcover: alk. paper)
Subjects: LCSH: Cooking (Herbs) | Nutrition. | Functional foods. | Naturopathy. | LCGFT: Cookbooks.
Classification: LCC TX819.H4 .B3885 2016 | DDC 641.6/57—dc23
LC record available at http://lccn.loc.gov/2015037838

Lovingly dedicated to my truly wonderful sister,
Leslie Horton Roberts

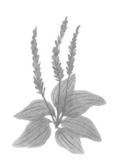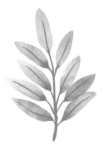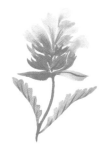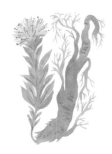

CONTENTS

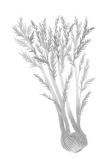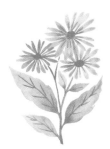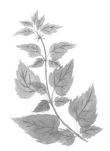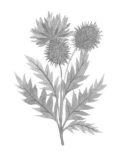

PART THREE **HEALING FOODS**

FOREWORD

THE KITCHEN HEARTH has long been the center of healing for common illnesses. Mothers, grandmothers, and other family members were on the front lines of restoring health within the family, and nourishing soups, herbal teas, elixirs, and syrups were their first and most obvious tools for healing and promoting the well-being of all.

Healing began to shift away from the hearth in the Middle Ages as people became fascinated with heroic, and often dangerous, interventions such as bloodletting and mercury medicines. Many people looked to outside experts instead of kitchen medicine, and their respect for home remedies decreased. By 1900 aspirin had been patented, and some decades later, antibiotics were widely available.

At the turn of the twentieth century, old-fashioned medicine from the hearth was no longer sought after in most of the United States. Pharmaceutical pills and "healthy living through science" became the norm. Even nutritious home cooking gave way to boxed foods and harmful manufactured substances such as margarine and corn syrup.

However, when we stepped away from kitchen medicine, we gave up power over our health. Instead of chicken soup and onion poultices, we turned to office visits and immune-suppressing medications that often do more harm than good.

Fortunately, we are beginning to see the errors of our ways. We are realizing that the key to health doesn't lie in a pill, and that food taken directly from the earth is our most powerful preventive medicine. We can re-empower ourselves and our families to proactively care for our own well-being.

The Healing Kitchen by Holly Bellebuono inspires us to reclaim kitchen medicine—to lovingly create delicious meals and potent herbal medicines to prevent and address common illnesses. There are many herbal recipe books available that make use of alcohol extractions, glycerin, witch hazel, and other store-bought menstruums, but the creations made this way best address acute situations. With *The Healing Kitchen,* Holly reminds us that our foundational health and nourishment should come from herbs and foods stewed on the kitchen hearth, and that love and community are powerful ingredients in our health and healing.

I encourage you to not only read this book but put it into action. Create these recipes. Offer them to your friends and family with love, and remember the powerful healing that comes from the hearth.

–Rosalee de la Forêt
Twisp, Washington
February 2015

INTRODUCTION

As a handcrafter, I spent my teenage years and my twenties making all sorts of functional art: pine needle baskets, quilts, soapstone jewelry, sewn clothes, wheel-thrown bowls and pottery. It was a way to nourish my creative side and experiment with handcrafting arts of all sorts—especially those prevalent in the North Carolina mountains where I grew up. As I delved into the lore and traditions of herbal medicine (another functional art), I learned to make healing remedies, a handcraft that combines the beauty of plants and flowers with the practical function of medicine and healing. Making herbal medicines allowed me to put my abundant garden harvest and meadow forage to excellent use. I made tinctures, salves, liniments, and syrups—all sorts of remedies that supported my growing family and kept us healthy.

It was only a hop and a jump, of course, to creating herbal remedies that were really foods—relying less on the grain-alcohol-based tinctures necessary for acute illnesses and putting my energy and time into making nourishing foods and drinks that support health and prevent illness. In other words, thinking ahead and being proactive.

Although I'm not a trained chef or even a cook by any means, for years I had been making homemade granola, yogurt, infused vinegars, oils, soups, and more. When I learned to include nutrient-packed edible and medicinal herbs in these meals and treats, it made that time in the kitchen all the more meaningful.

Taking herbal healing into the kitchen gives me the chance to care for others (in a delicious and nutritious way), but also to practice self-care, that slippery art that is seldom mastered but always sought. Extending my love of herbal crafting to creating nourishing foods that feed the soul has given me the opportunity to renew myself with every soup, broth, tea, and snack.

The kitchen, formerly an intimidating space for me, has become an extension of both my garden and my medicine cabinet—the epicenter of messy but creative experiments that help keep my family healthy and provide a respite from daily chores. I'm very lucky because my husband and daughter love to cook—they'll spend hours in the kitchen crafting delicious meals with chef-like enthusiasm, making mouthwatering gourmet entrées and keeping us well fed and healthy. But there is much more to a healing kitchen than main courses: when you learn to use edible and medicinal herbs, every snack, beverage, and condiment that you put in your body is a tasty opportunity to nourish, protect, and revitalize yourself and those you love.

Since I am no kitchen elf myself, I've designed and chosen recipes that are quick and easy. Many of them are in bulk amounts, so that the goodies you prepare—such as delicious and healing herbal salts, vinegars, stocks, powder blends, and drink blends—can be made in a large batch and stored. Then you can enjoy them again and again, knowing that with each serving you are not only indulging in the rich and robust flavors of the garden but also nourishing your body and mind with micronutrients and other herbal properties that uplift and support.

In addition, it was important to me that *The Healing Kitchen* be a collaborative effort. This is why, in addition to my own recipes, you'll find delicious contributions from nearly two dozen chefs, well-known authors, culinary artists, and herbalists from around the country. Their nourishing creations help round out this collection with imaginative ways to use culinary and medicinal herbs in the kitchen, and I hope you enjoy them.

FOOD AS MEDICINE

Why do herbs make our foods healthier? Our herbal *materia medica* is full of safe phytochemicals that support the work of the body and the mind and make us stronger and healthier. We eat vegetables for their minerals and vitamins, and we use herbal medicines to ease headaches, relieve muscle tension, strengthen the cardiovascular system, and build strong bones, so the goal of *The Healing Kitchen* is to combine these plant resources to create simultaneously nutritious and healing foods.

These recipes explore the bounty of the garden (and the health food store and farmer's market) using a wide variety of edible traditional healing herbs. We'll get creative with flavorful medicinal herbs, including berries (hawthorn, elderberry, and goji berry), seeds (especially plantain, fennel, chia, and lamb's-quarter), flowers (red clover, violet, hibiscus, and calendula), and leaves (nettles, hyssop, lemon balm, and many more), combining them with healthy grains, such as amaranth, oats, and millet; fats, such as avocados and butter; and even healthy meats, which we'll use to make hearty bone broths and main dishes.

Most of the herbs featured in the beverages, snacks, and dishes in this book have been used for centuries across the world for supporting the nervous system, strengthening the cardiovascular network, improving memory and clarity, and providing energy. They are revered herbal medicines from Western herbal traditions, Traditional Chinese Medicine, and the ancient Indian philosophy of Ayurveda, and they've survived not only because they are vital medicines for healing the sick but also because they are preventive, nourishing foods that shine in the culinary traditions of these world cultures.

Some spices, such as turmeric, are traditionally used to add flavor to and preserve dishes, such as curries in Indian cuisine. In Ayurvedic medicine, this same herb is used to relieve inflammatory illnesses, and in Western herbal medicine turmeric is valued to ease sore muscles and arthritis. Now, new research is showing how this favorite kitchen spice is showing promise as a treatment for Alzheimer's disease, and its use in *The Healing Kitchen* reflects this herb's versatility, flavor, color, and tradition.

THE BENEFITS OF AN HERBAL, HEALING KITCHEN

You may know that some herbs are called adaptogens—these help our bodies adapt to stress and are used to help us recover from anxiety, fear, or nerve-wracking experiences. Herbs such as ashwagandha, violet, nettles, rhodiola, and mint can be considered tonics that, used over time, help balance the way our bodies and mind deal with stress. You may also know that some herbs are called nervines—these help support our nervous system to relax or sleep well. There are also herbs that support the cardiovascular and digestive systems, helping the body perform at its peak. For centuries, people not only have used cinnamon, ginger, and other spices to coax incredible flavor out of their favorite foods but also have taken advantage of their warming properties to stimulate healthy circulation.

But you don't need an education in herbal medicine to enjoy these recipes and get the most from these delicious foods. Each recipe is designed to be easy to use in both city and country kitchens as well as healthy and healing for all ages. With these recipes, we will play with the abundance of healing herbs in a wide variety of dishes and drinks, allowing their flavors to sparkle while appreciating their subtle healing effects on our minds, bodies, and spirits.

Within these pages, you'll find easy instructions for using common and healing herbs in a wide variety of familiar foods: yogurt and milk, tea and chai, salsa and dips, even delicious homemade pastas and protein-rich grain salads. You'll also discover tips on making these daily foods work for you, such as sipping fennel broth when you have a cold or adding soothing herbs to hot milk to help you sleep at night. And almost every herb is described in detail, in more than seventy convenient sidebars, making learning about their benefits easy while you're mixing and preparing them in the kitchen.

AN INVITATION TO YOU

If you've always wanted to add more healing herbs to your cooking—or if you're new to cooking and would like to learn to make healthy, nourishing meals, snacks, beverages, and more—let this book be your welcoming guide. Feel free to experiment with fresh herbs that grow near you, using these recipes as the base for your creative expression.

Most of the recipes in this book are low-sugar or sugar-free and are created with ultimate nourishment and healing in mind; they are meant to be enjoyed over and over, to support and nourish you from the inside out throughout the year. Look for special icons throughout the book that indicate the benefits of each recipe: energizing, digestive support, heart support, stress support, nourishing and nutritious, calming, immune support, promotes clarity and memory, refreshing, and iron-rich.

From my garden and kitchen to yours, may this book be your guide to a healthy, delicious, messy, creative, fun-filled, and healing herbal culinary adventure!

RECIPE ICONS

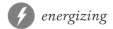 *energizing*

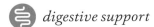 *digestive support*

heart support

stress support

nourishing

calming

immune support

clarity & memory

refreshing

iron-rich

THE HEALING HERBS PANTRY

IT'S TIME TO BREAK AWAY FROM SPINACH! There are so many delicious alternatives that offer great flavor as well as calcium, iron, and vitamins. And as we explore nourishing greens for our salads and sautés, we can also explore healing herbs for our salsas, chais, smoothies, crackers, soups, broths, breads, and even main dishes. From ashwagandha to zingiber, all the herbs in this book are nutritious edibles, and they all offer some kind of healing benefit.

Use fennel in your salt! It makes for an attractive and colorful blend that adds a bit of the unusual to your fish and chicken dinners (see Kitchen Digestive Spice Blend, page 21). Steep garlic scapes or bulbs in your vinegar: it's fun and delicious and gives you a bit of immune support when you're feeling under the weather (see Strong Garlic Vinegar, page 26). Best of all, once you make these recipes, you'll have some on hand for a long time: make the salt and vinegar when you have time, then keep them on your shelf or in your pantry to use whenever you like. There are so many easy ways to get healing herbs into your diet.

The recipes in this book include common garden herbs, such as rosemary, sage, thyme, oregano, violets, and lavender, as well as slightly unusual garden herbs, such as hyssop, bee balm, roses, and borage. I've also drawn from common meadow herbs that are readily found around the country, such as nettles, rose hips, dandelion, and burdock, as well as herbs that must generally be purchased at a well-stocked market, such as ashwagandha, rhodiola, and licorice. Investing in a few ounces of each of these and the other herbs in this book will be well worth the effort, as you'll use them again and again in the recipes. Refer to the sidebars to learn how each herb acts in the body to benefit you.

PLANT PARTS FOR KITCHEN USE

For the herbs we eat, we harvest certain parts of the plant for food, just as we do with common vegetables. For instance, we eat the leaves of nettles, catnip, and violets. We eat the seeds of fennel, plantain, and caraway. We use the roots of ginger and turmeric and the stem of angelica. Flowers are of particular value and can be used in many recipes: roses, violets, fennel, and elder are a few of the many beautiful blossoms that we can feature in medicinal recipes. Plan to use fresh herbs most of the time; to save some for later, refer to the next section for instructions on drying and storing your herbs.

Become familiar with a variety of healing herbs. One of the joys of cooking from *The Healing Kitchen* is expanding and enhancing your knowledge and understanding of the green plants that sustain us.

HARVESTING AND DRYING HERBS

If you are blessed with an abundance of angelica or a lot of lemon balm, you'll want to process it and store it properly so you can continue to use it after its growing season has passed. I've included recipes using both fresh and dried herbs, which in some cases must be ground. If you have access to a garden, a windowsill, or a bay window, you'll be able to grow many of the herbs to use fresh. Most can also be found at a farmer's market, health food store, or well-stocked grocery.

If you will be harvesting leafy herbs yourself, do it the day you plan to use them: snip off whole stems with leaves attached, and stand them up in a glass of water until ready to use. Also use purchased fresh herbs the same day. For dried herbs, whether purchased or dried at home, plan to use them within twelve months (use herb powders or ground spices within six months).

Generally, harvest herbs in midmorning, after any dew has dried but before the heat of the day sets in. To harvest the aerial, or aboveground, parts, snap them off cleanly with your fingers or snip them with scissors or clippers. Harvest from areas that have not been sprayed with chemicals of any kind and away from roadsides. There is generally no need to wash leaves, flowers, stems, or fruits.

You can easily dry most fresh leaves, flowers, and other aerial parts on a screen or on a table spread with newspapers. Set up your drying surface out of the sun, and make sure it's well ventilated. Dark attics with open windows work well, as do shady porches. Leave the leaves and flowers whole to dry them. If drying outdoors, a second screen can be set on top of lightweight herbs to keep them from blowing away in the wind. You can also use an electric dehydrator, but I've found that my quantity of herbs is usually far too much to fit on the little dehydrator shelves. I've also seen herbalists dry herbs in the propped-open trunk of their car. A shelf in a sunroom or greenhouse works well, as long as it is shady; when exposed to sunlight, herbs will quickly lose their color as well as their potency.

When harvesting roots, dig them up carefully and brush the dirt off with your fingers or a stiff brush. If storing the roots, place them in a paper bag or a box of straw or paper shavings. If using immediately, wash with an outdoor hose or in the sink, scrubbing vigorously and rinsing thoroughly. Pat dry. If you plan on drying them, slice the roots immediately, then spread them out on your screens or newspaper. Be sure to chop them into the shape or size you'll want as the final product, because once dry, they cannot easily be chopped again.

STORING HERBS

Dried herbs are so pretty, I've been tempted to store mine in clear glass jars so I can see them. Unfortunately, I've learned they inevitably fade, turning pale and losing their vibrant characteristics. It's better to store them in an airtight plastic bag, such as a Ziploc bag, wrapped inside another plastic bag for good measure, or in a paper grocery bag. It's not ideal, but it works. When stored in a plastic bag, they can be frozen for up to six months. The best method is to dry the herbs until they are crispy and then seal them in plastic using a vacuum-sealer machine that suctions out the air and creates an airtight seal. Whatever method you choose, be sure to label the bag clearly with the name of the herb, the date of harvest, and the date of storing.

When you make a salt, vinegar, or oil, however, you can put it into one of your favorite jars or bottles and store it right on the countertop. You'll be much more likely to use it there than if stored in the dark depths of the pantry!

STORING POWDERED HERBS

Whether you've ground your own dried herbs or purchased herb powders, store them in a dark, dry place. Make sure they are labeled. If you will not be using a particular powdered herb often, store it in a tightly sealed plastic bag away from moisture, either in a dark pantry or in the freezer. If you will be using an herb frequently, you can place it in a dark-glass jar and store it on a shelf within easy reach.

START WHERE YOU ARE

YOU DON'T NEED TO BE A CHEF to create tasty and nourishing goodies in your kitchen; cooking with herbs is fun and worthwhile regardless of your experience or culinary talent. Because these herb-inspired recipes tangibly benefit your physical and mental health, they make working in the kitchen that much more meaningful. No matter what your culinary experience has been, you can use these herbs to enhance your enjoyment of both cooking and eating. And don't let herbs intimidate you—most are very forgiving, and you don't need to worry too much about exact measurements. Let your taste buds be your guide, and treat most of these herbs as normal foods (that happen to have the power to excite, inspire, and deeply nourish you).

MAKE EVERY SNACK COUNT

In between meals, I like to nibble. I find that I feel best when I nibble and graze on something healthy and satisfying, such as Caraway Crackers (page 176) or Salsa Verde (page 166). I also like to drink herbal teas because they often help me feel satiated without the need to consume a lot of empty carbs or sugary snacks, especially when I let the herbal teas steep a long time to develop a robust, satisfying flavor; try the Deep Rooibos Chai on page 103, a nourishing drink that's perfect for nighttime when it's too late to eat food.

The trick to getting the most out of these recipes is to appreciate how beautiful, colorful, and appealing to the senses these healing and rejuvenating herbs really are. They are lovely growing in the garden, stunning packed in a basket, and attractive bottled on the countertop in the many festive preparations featured in these pages. Many of these recipes are designed to yield a substantial amount (of seasoned salt, granola, or dry tea blend, for example) so that they will be ready for you when you want them. Make a fresh batch of granola on the weekend so you can enjoy it all week, and prepare a tea blend from the dried herbs you harvested, so you can enjoy their flavor—and healing benefits—throughout the winter.

Whether you like the subtle, delicate flavors of Rose Petal Rice Pudding (page 221) or the bold, robust taste of Yang Vinegar (page 30) and Strong Garlic Oil (page 36), let herbs be the highlight of your kitchen experience. Enjoy these nourishing foods throughout your day—from breakfast to lunch to dinner and everything in between—knowing that herbs are supporting and building a better you.

A SOULFUL PRACTICE

I teach my herbalism students that I believe it's the connection that counts the most—that special relationship between a client and an herbalist, and between people and plants. Cultivating a strong connection with healing herbs in your kitchen is a meaningful way to be present and to appreciate what these plants have to offer. Through this delicious and soulful practice, you will grow as a cook, as a healer, and as an integral part of the greater community in which we are all connected.

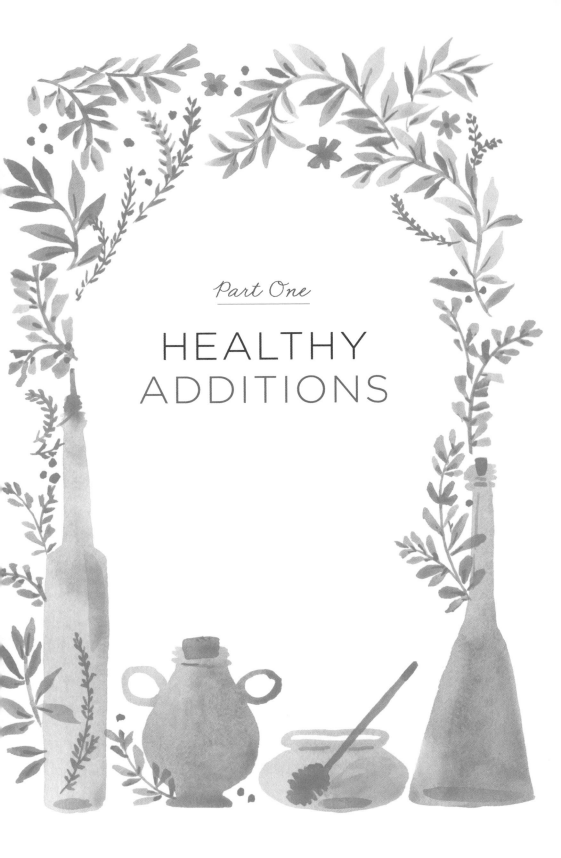

Part One

HEALTHY
ADDITIONS

1

GOMASIOS, HERB-INFUSED FINISHING SALTS, AND SPICE BLENDS

THEY SAY VARIETY IS THE SPICE OF LIFE, and in the kitchen this is certainly true. A good herbal kitchen is a playhouse of tastes, textures, and fragrances, and the joyful cook can experiment to her heart's desire. Banish the plain canister of iodized salt from your shelf! Instead, explore using your own salt blends and mixes made with salts from around the world combined with herbs from your garden, from the wild, and from the sea.

These blends can be made in bulk and stored in glass jars with tight-fitting lids. (I love glass jars; in fact, I have something of an obsession with them! Luckily, it's an herbalist's prerogative to own dozens of glass jars in different shapes and sizes.) For salts and seasoning blends, small wide-mouthed jars are ideal because they allow you to reach in to take a pinch or to use a small scoop or attractive hand-carved spoon. Many chefs place a saltcellar on the table for their guests; speckled with dulse, parsley, fennel, and more, yours will be doubly beautiful served this way.

Making blends is an activity where children can shine. Let them participate in the scooping and measuring, knowing that it's hard to go wrong with these blends. It's fun to let little hands help out, especially if you'll be harvesting the herbs yourself and then drying them before adding them to the salts. Children can participate in the whole process: picking the leaves, spreading them out to dry, crumbling them up, and then helping you measure and mix. At mealtime they can sprinkle a pinch over their plate and enjoy the fantastically tasty seasoning they made.

As long as the ingredients stay dry, these mixes will last indefinitely.

GOMASIO

Gomasio is a traditional Japanese blend of sea salt and toasted sesame seeds, resulting in a rich and textured seasoning. Rich in calcium, iron, and other trace minerals, sea salt and sesame seeds combine well with seaweeds and herbs to produce powerfully nutritious—and delicious—blends. Sprinkle gomasio on meat and fish, scrambled eggs, and salad greens with olive oil and vinegar. Keep your gomasio right on the table in an attractive saltcellar or dish so it can be enjoyed frequently.

Simple Gomasio by Kate Gilday

 iron-rich | YIELDS ABOUT ¼ CUP

"Many years ago," says herbalist Kate Gilday, "I began to prepare a simple gomasio with sea salt and raw sesame seeds. I would toast the seeds, cool them, and then grind them with sea salt. I loved the taste and would use this condiment on rice and other grains, as well as on popcorn, on vegetables, or in soups." Kate suggests trying this Simple Gomasio recipe first, and then adding a wild green or seaweed, one at a time, to gradually create more complex recipes, "so you can choose your ingredients wisely."

¼ cup sesame seeds

1 teaspoon salt of your choice, such as sea salt or pink Himalayan salt

Heat a cast iron skillet over medium heat. Pour in the sesame seeds and lightly toast them, stirring frequently, until they are fragrant, 3 to 5 minutes.

Add the salt and cook, stirring continuously, for another 30 seconds. Transfer the mixture into a bowl and let cool. Using a coffee grinder or mortar and pestle, pulse or grind to the desired consistency, being careful not to over-grind the mixture into a paste or seed butter. Store in a labeled glass jar.

Wild Greens Gomasio by Kate Gilday

 iron-rich | YIELDS ABOUT ¼ CUP

Traditional gomasio can be made more interesting and versatile using a wide variety of local herbs. Kate notes, "As time went by, I learned the value of sea vegetables and began adding a bit of dulse or kelp to the mix. Then came my study of herbs and wild greens, and I began adding dried nettle leaf and occasionally milk thistle seed." Both nettles and sesame seeds are high in calcium, making this a mineral-rich addition to sprinkle on pasta dishes, scrambled eggs, sautéed fish, and steamed vegetables.

¼ **cup sesame seeds**

1 tablespoon dulse or kelp flakes

1 tablespoon crushed dried nettles

½ **teaspoon salt of your choice, such as sea salt or pink Himalayan salt**

Heat a cast iron skillet over medium heat. Pour in the sesame seeds and lightly toast them, stirring frequently, until they are fragrant, 3 to 5 minutes. Add the salt, seaweed, and nettles and cook, stirring continuously, for another 30 seconds. Transfer the mixture into a bowl and let cool. Using a coffee grinder or mortar and pestle, pulse or grind to the desired consistency, being careful not to overgrind the mixture into a paste or seed butter. Store in a labeled glass jar.

Wildflower Gomasio

 nourishing | YIELDS ABOUT ¼ CUP

Colorful and pretty—boasting pink, golden, and bright red petals—this blend can be sprinkled on pasta with garlic and oil and on fresh green salads. Calendula has long been used as an immune-support herb, and bee balm, which is in the mint family, lends its lovely minty aroma to this tasty blend. Shred the flowers by tearing them apart with your fingers, coarsely pulling the petals from the flower head, which can be discarded. Use only the petals in these recipes.

¼ **cup sesame seeds**

2 tablespoons shredded dried red clover flowers

1 tablespoon shredded dried calendula flowers

1 tablespoon shredded dried bee balm flowers

1 teaspoon salt of your choice, such as sea salt or pink Himalayan salt

Heat a cast iron skillet over medium heat. Pour in the sesame seeds and lightly toast them, stirring frequently, until they are fragrant, 3 to 5 minutes. Add the dried flowers and salt and cook, stirring continuously, for another 30 seconds. Pour and scrape the mixture onto a plate and let cool. Using a coffee grinder or mortar and pestle, quickly pulse or grind the mixture to the desired consistency. Store in a labeled glass jar.

FINISHING SALTS

I've always been enamored of small saltcellars packed with colorful and mysterious dried herbs and spices that are crushed together with coarse sea salt. Harvested from the sea, this salt is rich in minerals, and its depth of flavor complements a variety of herbal flavors. Combining herbs and salt is an imaginative way to create seasonings in the kitchen, and I was thrilled to find the work of Juliet Blankespoor, the author and director of the Chestnut School of Herbal Medicine, who is doing exactly that. Says Juliet:

> Herb-infused finishing salts are a delightful alchemy between earth and sea, plant and mineral. . . . Surprisingly easy to con-jure up and beautiful to behold, herbal salts provide an easy way to preserve excess fresh culinary herbs. They are called "finishing salts" because they are added to a dish after it is prepared. However, many of these salt blends are perfect for adding to marinades and dressings. Or they can be rubbed on meats and seafood before roasting or panfrying. I enjoy finish-ing salts on popcorn, eggs, and to flavor goat cheese spreads.

You'll need a food processor or coffee grinder, but other equipment is unnecessary. For Juliet's recipes that follow, you'll be combining fresh herbs with salt in roughly equal proportions and then drying the mixture, keeping in mind that the more fresh herbs you include, the longer the

SEAWEEDS

Alaria spp., *Hizikia fusiformis,* and other species

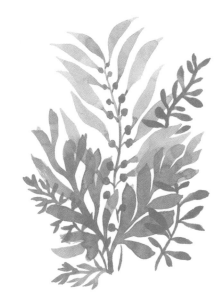

Delicious and versatile, seaweeds are extremely high in carotenes, calcium, potassium, magnesium, sodium, silicon, selenium, and more, yet they may contain damaging minerals, including arsenic, tin, nickel, chloride, and lead; use common sense when consuming them, limiting intake to no more than 1 to 2 tablespoons of crumbled dried seaweed per day. Kelp, dulse, and hijiki can support those with fatigue, muscle debility, and nervous exhaustion. Include seaweeds in small amounts in vinegars, sautés, dishes with steamed greens, and broths, and eat them raw as a snack.

CALENDULA

Calendula officinalis

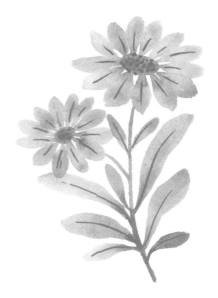

Calendula, commonly called pot marigold, is a favorite among herbalists for its beauty and quick action. Frequently used as a topical remedy for wounds, cuts, and burns, and especially useful for treating eczema, psoriasis, and topical yeast infections, calendula is also used internally to treat internal yeast and fungal infections such as *Candida albicans*. Very mild yet effective, calendula is prized as a remedy for infants, young children, and those with sensitive skin. It is nourishing for dry skin and helpful for healing rashes, damaged skin, and scarring. True marigolds, *Tagetes* spp. (that is, various species in the *Tagetes* genus), are also highly nourishing and can be used interchangeably with calendula for skin rashes and itching. Eat calendula petals raw in salads, sprinkle them on rice and grain dishes, and use them in syrups, elixirs, and vinegars. Because calendula is quite bitter, use it sparingly in herbal teas and smoothies.

blend will take to dry. You can also use dried herbs instead of fresh: Juliet recommends using one-quarter the amount of herbs called for in the recipe; simply omit the drying step and store the blend in an airtight glass jar.

To achieve a spectrum of flavors, colors, and textures, experiment with different herbs and a variety of salts from around the world. You will be rewarded with a versatile and mineral-rich condiment full of lasting flavor.

Dusky Desert Finishing Salt
by Juliet Blankespoor

YIELDS ABOUT 1¼ CUP

Highlighting juniper berries and sage, this is a pungent blend that is especially good on chicken dishes, on roasted potatoes, and in stuffing. "You can also add it to olive oil and vinegar to create a flavorful salad dressing," suggests Juliet, "or sprinkle it on sweet potato and black bean casseroles and burritos." It's also a great contrast to the sweetness of winter squash, and Juliet uses it as a bright garnish on squash bisque.

15 juniper berries

⅓ cup tightly packed fresh rosemary leaves (removed from stems)

1 teaspoon dried orange zest

3 tablespoons tightly packed whole sage leaves

1 cup coarse salt (pink Himalayan salt, black volcanic sea salt, and/or smoked sea salt)

2 teaspoons minced garlic

¼ teaspoon coarsely ground black pepper

Mash the juniper berries with a mortar and pestle, or use the side of a chef's knife to crush them against a cutting board. In a large bowl, combine the mashed juniper berries and the rest of the ingredients. Spread out the mixture on a serving tray or baking sheet and place in an area with good airflow. Allow the herbs to dry completely. Juliet suggests placing the trays on a table or countertop under a ceiling fan for 2 to 4 days. "The salt speeds up the drying process, simultaneously absorbing the flavor of the fresh herbs along with the moisture," she says.

Alternatively, use the oven method for quick drying: Preheat your oven to its lowest setting. Spread out the mixture on a baking sheet, place it in the oven, and prop open the door slightly with a long-handled wooden spoon. Allow the mixture to gently heat for several hours, stirring frequently, until the herbs are dry and crisp. Remove the baking sheet from the oven and allow the mixture to cool completely. Juliet warns that this method will allow some of the essential oils of the herbs to evaporate, thus decreasing their aroma and flavor, so favor the slow drying method if you have the time.

Once dried, store the blend in an airtight glass jar and grind as needed.

Lemon–White Sage Finishing Salts
by Juliet Blankespoor

YIELDS ABOUT 1 CUP

Together, lemon zest and sage make a memorable, sharp-and-tangy combination. "This is one of my favorite herb-infused finishing salts," says Juliet, "and it is delightful to prepare, as the aroma is so uplifting." She suggests adding it to Thanksgiving stuffing, chicken dishes, and roasted portobello mushrooms. Use either white sage (*Salvia apiana*) or garden sage (*Salvia officinalis*).

Handful of whole sage leaves

1 cup coarse pink Himalayan salt

2 tablespoons grated fresh lemon zest

In a medium bowl, combine all the ingredients. Follow the instructions for the Dusky Desert Finishing Salt, page 20.

Kitchen Digestive Spice Blend

 digestive support | YIELDS ABOUT 1 CUP

These time-honored garden herbs are digestive healers and have been favorites in Western cooking for centuries. Ginger adds a slight kick, and caraway imparts its strong flavor to make this a very tasty and surprising seasoning. Use this herb-loving salt to season a variety of dishes, from scrambled eggs to spring salads to steamed greens.

½ cup coarse sea salt

2 teaspoons fennel seeds

2 teaspoons dried chopped ginger (not ground ginger)

1 teaspoon dried chopped lemon peel

1 teaspoon coriander seeds

½ teaspoon caraway seeds

Put all the ingredients into a coffee grinder and pulse until the desired "grind" is reached; some of the fennel may remain whole. If you want it all finely ground, simply grind the fennel before adding the other ingredients. Store in a half-pint glass jar.

SPICE BLENDS

Combining a wide range of flavors in spice blends is part of the fun of herbal crafting. "Spices" are generally the fruits, seeds, and barks of strong-smelling aromatic plants, while herbs are generally the leaves and flowers. Spices and herbs combine well to create healthy and flavorful remedies and dishes, and there is no end to how you can use your imagination to make the most of them. Many spices have antibacterial properties, and many are warming and stimulate the circulatory system, which can make them valuable for those who are feeling fatigued or overcoming an illness. Every culture has its own history with certain spices and its own favorite combinations; experiment freely to discover your own go-to flavors. Keep your blends in an airtight jar right on the kitchen countertop to encourage using them often.

Za'atar Mix

 immune support | YIELDS ABOUT 1 CUP

Za'atar is an ancient and delicious blend of pungent thyme and oregano, tart and lemony sumac berries, and zesty and sweet spices. I am quite liberal with the salt in this recipe because it really brings out all the flavor of the herbs. In this recipe, I've drawn from the traditional heritage of Jordan and its multitude of versatile, oregano-based za'atar recipes. In particular, I drew inspiration from Princess Basma bint Ali of Jordan, who shared her family's recipe with me for my book *Women Healers of the World*. A popular Jordanian snack is warm, fresh-from-the-bakery *mangoosha* dipped into a flavorful olive oil sprinkled with za'atar; substitute a freshly baked baguette for the *mangoosha* for a wonderful treat. I also love tart-and-salty za'atar on my scrambled eggs in the morning or spread onto a baguette and eaten with hard cheese.

I harvest my own sumac berries in the autumn, and although the sumac gathered in the Middle East is slightly different from the American sumac species (which have smaller seeds), it's fine to use the fruits of our crimson-colored staghorn sumac in this recipe. To gather sumac berries, wait until the sumac-berry clusters, or "horns," are a deep, rich scarlet color (don't use white sumac berries, which indicate they are from the poison sumac plant); gently rub your finger on a few red berries and then lick your finger: you should taste a vibrant lemony flavor, indicating that the berries are ripe and ready. Snap off the entire horn and collect the horns in a paper bag; at home, strip the berries from the horns, dry them, and store them in an airtight container. Sumac berries are also available in specialty markets. When preparing the berries for za'atar, grind them very finely.

- 2 teaspoons sesame seeds
- 2 teaspoons dried wild thyme leaves
- 2 teaspoons crumbled dried marjoram leaves
- 2 teaspoons ground sumac berries
- 2 teaspoons crumbled dried oregano leaves
- 1 teaspoon cumin seeds
- 1 teaspoon coarse salt
- ½ teaspoon ground cinnamon, optional

In a cast iron skillet over medium-low heat, gently toast the sesame seeds until warm and fragrant, just a few minutes. Quickly transfer the seeds to a bowl and let cool. Add the thyme, marjoram, sumac, oregano, cumin, salt, and cinnamon and stir well to combine. Store in an airtight glass jar.

American Allspice Berry Seasoning
by Doug Elliott

American allspice berries from the *Lindera benzoin* tree are a prized flavoring ingredient much like the familiar allspice from Central and South America. I've heard this lovely smooth-leafed tree called "Indian spicebush," but most herbalists call it simply spicebush. To make "tea," traditional gatherers up and down the East Coast collect the twigs (milder) and the leaves (stronger). The herbalist and storyteller Doug Elliott uses the twigs to flavor wild game and the berries to flavor robust dishes. "It is particularly good in apple dishes, pastries, curries, and chutney," he says. I find a small amount of ground allspice makes a surprising but effective addition to tomato sauce, as well, and consider using your dried American allspice berries in one of the mulling spice blends in chapter 6.

Gather the berries when they are ripe (usually in September in the South, earlier in New England). Dry them in a food dehydrator, or spread them out in a thin single layer on a screen or table covered with newspaper and set in a well-ventilated area in the shade.

Once dried, store the berries in a labeled glass jar with a tight-fitting lid. Grind them in a food processor or, better yet, a coffee grinder, and use the powder as a flavoring the way you would allspice.

SUMAC

Rhus typhina and other species

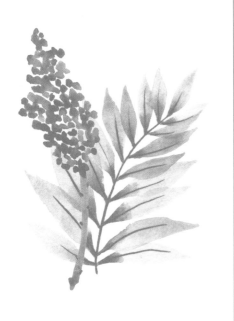

Tart and tangy, red sumac berries are a key ingredient in spicy za'atar mixes and sum-mer lemonades. I love to harvest sumac berries in the fall and make a pot of Sumac "Lemonade" (page 127). I also like to dry them, grind them with oregano, thyme, and salt, and sprinkle the blend over olive oil to create a traditional Middle Eastern bread-dipping oil. Harvest the entire head of berries, technically *drupes*, and place it in a pot of cool water for fresh lemon-ade, or spread several on newsprint in the shade to dry. Crumble dried sumac berries into chai blends, mulling spice blends, and herbal teas, or *tisanes*.

2

VINEGARS, OILS, AND PESTOS

MOST OF US USE VINEGARS AND OILS on a daily basis in our kitchens, but we may not realize that these "condiments" can be made much more potent and medicinally valuable than when they come off the shelf. Take a simple vinegar or a mild-flavored oil and steep some nutritious herbs in it: it becomes a vehicle of vibrant flavor, packed with minerals and vitamins. This process is called infusing, and it's one of my favorite ways to preserve the garden harvest and also create beautiful gifts. Stock your pantry with infused oils and vinegars that showcase the beauty of the garden harvest, and you'll be giving your body much-needed nutrients in every little way possible.

VINEGARS

Be choosy about your vinegars. Generally, leave white distilled vinegar on the shelf next to the washing machine—although it's good for making pickles, it's a strong, high-acid vinegar that's useful mostly as a household cleaner and disinfectant. Balsamic vinegar and red and white wine vinegars are great for salads, but for vinegar infused with herbs, choose a good organic, unpasteurized apple cider vinegar, preferably one that includes the "mother," which means it still has strains of the original fermenting solids in it, including proteins, enzymes, and stomach-healthy bacteria.

Many of these herbal vinegars work wonderfully in salad dressings. Simply combine three parts infused vinegar to one part oil. The herbal oils that follow pair especially well with these vinegars: see the chart on page 41 for recommended pairings.

How to Make an Herbal Vinegar

There are two ways to make infused vinegars: with or without heat. I prefer gently heating the vinegar (just barely to a simmer); this way it readily breaks down the cell walls of the plants I'm infusing, to draw the minerals out more efficiently. Be careful to not let the vinegar boil or even bubble: when it just reaches a simmer, pour it into a bottle or jar with your chosen herbs and cap it with a cork or a plastic lid. (To use a metal lid, first cover the jar with wax paper or unbleached baking parchment, then screw on the lid; this will prevent the lid from rusting closed.)

Label your bottle or jar and place it on a dish on a shelf in a dark, cool space. Let it steep for at least two weeks and up to several months, shaking and tilting the jar occasionally. After steeping, strain the herbs out through a fine-mesh sieve and store in a clean bottle or jar. You can serve a clear vinegar, or just before serving you can add fresh herbs for a pretty presentation and a little fresh flavor. Use this vinegar on salads (combine three parts vinegar to one part oil), in a glass of water as a tonic, on steamed vegetables with salt and pepper, or with honey in elixir recipes (see chapter 4).

Strong Garlic Vinegar

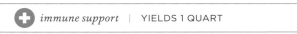 *immune support* | YIELDS 1 QUART

This is a wonderful way to get fresh, uncooked garlic into your diet. We know garlic as a food and a flavoring, but it's also a medicine. In herbal traditions raw garlic is often used to treat atherosclerosis and heart disease, to support the immune system against colds and viruses, to kill roundworms and other parasites, and even to support the immune system to fight cancer. To get more raw garlic in your daily diet, use this vinegar frequently—on salads, over steamed broccoli, kale, or spinach, or on sautéed Brussels sprouts. Or mix it with a little honey to create an elixir (see page 72).

- 1 quart apple cider vinegar
- 2 cups whole garlic cloves (about 30 to 40 cloves), peeled
- 2 cups fresh whole leaves or 10 to 12 sprigs of an herb of your choice (such as thyme, oregano, sage, and/or rosemary), optional

Gently warm the vinegar in a large saucepan over medium-low heat. Place the garlic cloves and herbs in a 1-quart glass jar and pour the warmed vinegar over them. Gently swirl the jar to release air bubbles, and cap tightly with a nonmetallic lid. Place the jar on a small dish to catch any liquid that may ooze out, and store in a cupboard or other dark place for at least 2 weeks and up to 6 months. Strain. (Save the preserved garlic to use in salads or pickle dishes.) Store the infused vinegar in a clean, labeled jar or bottle, and use within 2 years.

ROSEMARY

Rosmarinus officinalis

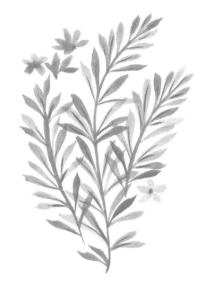

Highly aromatic rosemary is widely regarded as a prime healing aid and useful medicine both in the United States and throughout Europe. Commonly used as a culinary herb for its fragrance and pine-scented leaves, it is a very strong, warming remedy with overt actions on many systems of the body. Rosemary essential oil can be inhaled in steam baths for relief of upper respiratory congestion and lower respiratory infections; it readily opens nasal and bronchial passageways to ease breathing and relieve mucous congestion. It is a popular aromatherapy remedy for alertness, concentration, and wakefulness. Brewed as a *tisane*, or herbal "tea," it can be drunk in small amounts to support healthy blood pressure and mental clarity. Used in small quantities in syrups and elixirs, it gives a piney and robust flavor.

Minty Salad Vinegar

 clarity & memory | YIELDS 1 QUART

For a fresh, minty flavor on salads, these herbs are ideal. You'll be getting minerals and nutrients while enjoying a summery treat.

- 1 quart apple cider vinegar or white wine vinegar
- Handful of fresh hyssop leaves, chopped
- Handful of fresh mint leaves (any kind), chopped
- Handful of fresh lemon balm leaves, chopped
- 2 tablespoons chopped fresh summer or winter savory leaves, optional

Gently warm the vinegar in a large saucepan over medium-low heat. Place the herbs in a 1-quart glass jar and pour the warmed vinegar over them. Gently swirl the jar to release air bubbles, and cap tightly with a nonmetallic lid. Place the jar on a small dish to catch any liquid that may ooze out, and store in a cupboard or other dark place for at least 2 weeks and up to 6 months. Strain. Store the infused vinegar in a clean, labeled jar or bottle, and use within 2 years.

Green Nettle Vinegar

 iron-rich | YIELDS 1 QUART

Use fresh nettle leaves and stems for the most flavorful and nutritious vinegar. Combine this vinegar with olive oil for salads, or sprinkle it over steamed broccoli with salt and pepper.

- 1 quart apple cider vinegar or dark balsamic vinegar
- 4 cups chopped fresh nettle leaves and stems

Follow the instructions for Minty Salad Vinegar, above.

Deep-Toning Strengthening Vinegar

 iron-rich | YIELDS 1 QUART

One of the reasons I like to use vinegar is that it is ideal for drawing minerals out of herbs: for example, calcium, iron, and magnesium are easily extracted into vinegar and are therefore more easily assimilated by the body when ingested this way. The herbs used in this strengthening vinegar are mineral-rich and excellent for enriching and building blood in those with anemia or who have just had surgery.

　　1 quart apple cider vinegar

　　1 cup packed chopped fresh dandelion leaves

　　1 cup chopped fresh dandelion root (well washed)

　　1 cup chopped fresh burdock root (well washed)

　　½ cup chopped fresh gingerroot

　　½ cup packed chopped fresh heal-all leaves

　　½ cup marjoram

Follow the instructions for Minty Salad Vinegar, page 28.

Daily Vinegar

 refreshing | YIELDS 1 QUART

If you want to experiment and play with herbs in all their variety, this vinegar is the way to do it. It's a smorgasbord of taste, aroma, and color, and it will wake up any salad. Use this vinegar daily by the spoonful or as a dressing for all your raw or steamed vegetables and greens. Feel free to substitute different herbs and add other herbs and flowers to your heart's desire.

　　1 quart apple cider vinegar

　　1 cup fresh thyme or oregano leaves

　　1 cup chopped fresh nettle

　　2 cups fresh leaves and flowers of assorted herbs—
　　　　choose from the following:

　　　　Borage leaves and flowers

　　　　Fennel flowers, fronds, or seeds

Peeled garlic

Chickweed tops

Calendula flowers

Nasturtium flowers

Bay leaves

Lavender leaves and flowers

Rosemary leaves

Sage

Marjoram

Savory

Dill

Follow the instructions for Minty Salad Vinegar, page 28, and add a few fresh rosemary stems to the strained vinegar. Use within 2 years.

Yang Vinegar

 energizing | YIELDS 1 QUART

These herbs are strengthening, energizing herbs that invigorate. This type of energy is considered "yang" energy in Traditional Chinese Medicine, and it can be appreciated in the effects of a cayenne pepper: hot, dry, energizing. (Alternatively, "yin" energy is considered cool, wet, and relaxed.) People can use a boost of "yang" energy when they are nervous or fatigued, when the weather is cold, or when they are recovering from an illness. To get a burst of yang herbs, include hot and spicy herbs such as sage, peppermint, and wild sarsaparilla in this delicious vinegar and use it daily on salads, drizzled over steamed vegetables, or by the spoonful.

1 quart apple cider vinegar

1 cup nasturtium flowers

1 cup sage leaves

1 cup peppermint leaves

½ cup chopped wild sarsaparilla (*Aralia nudicaulis*) root (well washed), optional

Follow the instructions for Minty Salad Vinegar, page 28, and add fresh nasturtium flower to the strained vinegar, if desired. Use within 2 years.

HEAL-ALL (SELF-HEAL)

Prunella vulgaris

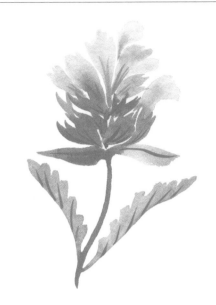

This lovely purplish green wildflower has long been a favorite in folk medicine and was historically considered a panacea, an herb that heals everything. Heal-all provides a gentle astringent effect that pairs nicely with stronger expectorants (such as coltsfoot) for respiratory congestion and excessive mucus. It offers enough mineral content to serve as a micronutrient-malnutrition tonic and can be used safely in infusions, rinses, and syrups.

WILD SARSAPARILLA

Aralia nudicaulis

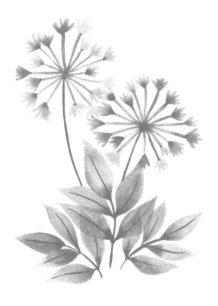

An herb with tremendous "yang" energy, wild sarsaparilla provides stimulating and warming energy to all extremities and to the core of the body, giving a "lift" and a sense of vascular excitement without caffeine. It is useful as a male tonic, as well as for debilitated conditions of weakness and lethargy and nervous exhaustion. A "cousin" of ginseng, this plant is not at risk and is native to North America. While it makes an excellent alcohol tincture, it performs equally well in an infusion or decoction, infused in vinegar, and as a honey.

Grape Leaf Vinegar by Robin Rose Bennett

 heart support | YIELDS 1 PINT

The main mission of our tiniest blood vessels, our capillaries, is to be a bridge between our veins and arteries, so they need to be permeable, teaches herbalist Robin Rose Bennett. Capillaries are so thin and fragile that they break easily as we age, especially because most of us spend too much time sitting in chairs and with our legs crossed. Grape plants used internally and/or externally will strengthen the elasticity of those hair-thin capillaries and reduce breakage, Robin says: "I love using grape leaves, vines, and tendrils, both internally and topically, for enhancing circulation of blood and improving the health of the blood vessels with their array of antioxidant bioflavonoids." She uses grape tea or tincture as a pain reliever and anti-inflammatory, and to help with leg pain and varicosities, including hemorrhoids. Fresh leaf poultices applied directly to the veins are beneficial for shrinking swollen veins, as are applications of grape leaf vinegar. This was confirmed for Robin when her father used the remedy for varicose veins:

> My dad had varicose veins for a long time and his legs would tire, but years later, when he began to have so much pain at night that it was keeping him from sleeping and even sometimes waking him up, he found a doctor who performed surgery on one leg, and planned to do the other. They needed to wait several months for his healing, however, before the second surgery. We added grape leaf into his herbal-care practices, and after several months the surgeon agreed with my dad's assessment that he no longer needed the surgery.

Robin suggests using grape internally and externally to help any tissue where blood is leaking from the vessels and causing purplish blotches on the skin, and also to help heal purple, black, and yellow bruises. She notes that you can apply this vinegar externally on the skin over swollen veins and broken capillaries: rub a few drops into the affected area several times daily using your fingers or a cotton ball. You can also use this vinegar internally to help heal inflamed joints: sprinkle it on salads, over cooked greens, and in sauces. You can add a teaspoon to water and simply drink it, or it can be mixed with an equal amount of honey and ingested. Take 1 teaspoon one to three times daily.

1 cup chopped fresh grape leaves, vines, and tendrils

1 to 1½ cups apple cider vinegar

Place the herbs in a 1-pint glass jar and pour the vinegar over them, filling the jar to the top. Wait a few minutes for it to settle, then top the jar off one more time and cap. Place on a dish in a cabinet or other dark place and allow it to sit, undisturbed, for at least 2 weeks. Strain. Store the infused vinegar in a clean, labeled jar or bottle, and use within 2 years.

Vinegar of the Four Thieves

 immune support | YIELDS 1 QUART

This is one of many variations on the legendary remedy supposedly used by French thieves during the bubonic plague. Alternate legends abound, indicating the vinegar was created by thieves in France or England, in the fourteenth century or in the seventeenth century, before pillaging or after arrest, and possibly by a man named Richard Forthave. No one knows the true origin of the formula itself, which also hops around from ingredient to ingredient. However, most formulas contain many of the common Mediterranean herbs, some bitter herbs, and added camphor powder. In addition to the herbs used in this recipe, popular herbs include oregano, horehound, marjoram, meadowsweet, cloves, wormwood, camphor, and rosemary. All the old recipes use a base of vinegar—made from white wine, red wine, or apple cider.

This particular immune-system-supporting version has an intense, deep flavor with a hint of bitterness, perfect for mixing with honey for an elixir (see page 72) or for topping robust foods such as steamed broccoli or nettles. All herbs are used fresh.

1 quart apple cider vinegar

1 cup thyme

½ cup sage

½ cup lavender

½ cup savory

½ cup angelica

½ **cup rue**

5 garlic cloves, peeled and bruised

Follow the instructions for making Minty Salad Vinegar, page 28, and add peeled garlic cloves to the strained vinegar, if desired. Use within 2 years.

Bright Vinegar for Colds

 immune support | YIELDS 1 QUART

Support your immune system with daily teaspoons of this intense, heady, and aromatic vinegar. My children are vinegar fanatics and regularly sip this vinegar from a spoon all winter long. They love the tangy flavor and intensity in the mouth. Make this vinegar in the harvest season of autumn so it's ready for you to take at the first sign of a cold or the flu; mix a teaspoon of the vinegar in a small cup of water and sip either cold or hot.

2 to 3 cups apple cider vinegar

1 cup dried elderberries

1 cup fresh thyme leaves

1 cup packed chopped fresh cleavers

½ **cup chopped onion**

½ **cup chopped fresh garlic**

¼ **cup chopped fresh horseradish root or prepared horseradish from a jar**

Follow the instructions for making Minty Salad Vinegar, page 28.

Fruit Vinegar for Salads

 refreshing | YIELDS 1 QUART

Fruit and vinegar were made for each other. All sorts of fruits go well steeped in vinegar, and there are many things you can do with the result: heat it with sugar and drizzle on ice cream for a punchy, zingy topping; sprinkle it over a soft cheese and eat with crackers or focaccia; mix it with honey to create an elixir; or drizzle it onto steamed bell peppers or asparagus.

Use fresh berries whenever possible, and experiment with various vinegars for the right balance of sweet and tart.

1 quart white wine or apple cider vinegar

1 cup fresh elderberries, or ½ cup dried

2 cups pitted and chopped fresh beach plums or any type of cherry or plum

1 cup fresh or frozen cranberries

½ cup dried schizandra berries or goji berries

1 cup raw cane sugar or honey, optional

Follow the instructions for Minty Salad Vinegar, page 28. After the vinegar has steeped and the solids have been strained with a fine-mesh sieve, gently whisk the optional sugar or honey into the vinegar, gently reheating the vinegar if necessary. Store the infused vinegar in a clean, labeled jar or bottle, and use within 2 years.

OILS

Drizzled over baked fish or sautéed vegetables, mixed with basil for pesto, or blended with vinegar for salad dressing, infused oils lend their strong flavor to many dishes. For your oil base, choose from a variety of thin or thick oils, including walnut, olive, sunflower, sesame, sweet almond, and anything else that appeals to you. Purchase oils that have been cold pressed, not heat processed or extracted with chemicals. Plan to use these infused oils in salad dressings and drizzled over vegetables, but use caution if cooking with them: the heat may destroy some of the nutritional benefits of the herbs.

How to Make an Herbal Oil

It's easy to infuse oil with nutritious and tasty herbs. Choose dried herbs and spices, or harvest fresh herbs and then wilt them by spreading them on a sheet of newspaper or a screen. The herbs and all the equipment that come in contact with the oil should be completely dry, as moisture can quickly lead to the formation of mold or dangerous food toxins, ruining the oil.

STOVE-TOP METHOD. While the sit-on-the-shelf folk method works well for infusing oils with herbs—especially when the oil will be used topically or in a bath—the best process for crafting a safe, edible herbal oil begins on the stove top. Place the herbs and the oil of choice into a clean, very dry glass canning jar and place the jar into a saucepan filled roughly one-quarter full with water. Alternatively, place the herbs and the oil into the saucepan directly, using no jar or water, but keep the heat very low and stir frequently. Using either method, gently heat the pan, keeping the water or oil just below a simmer, for about 2 hours or according to each recipe's instructions. When stirring, be sure to use a dry spoon, scrape with a dry spatula, and strain with a dry strainer or dry hands.

Remove the pan from the heat and allow the oil to cool. When it is cool enough to handle, strain the oil, squeezing the herbs with your hands to extract as much as possible—it's messy, but it gets much more oil out of the herbs than pressing through a sieve alone.

Strain the infused oil into a clean, dry, and labeled bottle or jar. Refrigerate the oil immediately and store it for up to one week.

Strong Garlic Oil

 immune support | YIELDS 1 QUART

Use this to flavor foods with a lovely, fresh, intense garlic flavor. I like it drizzled onto steamed broccoli or fresh pasta. Because oils infused with garlic and other vegetables can harbor botulism spores, be sure to follow the recipe carefully and store the finished oil in the refrigerator. Use it within 1 week. Alternatively, this can be rubbed topically onto sore muscles to help relieve pain.

> 20 to 30 garlic cloves, peeled
> ½-inch piece of fresh gingerroot, chopped
> 1 tablespoon fresh thyme leaves, or 1 teaspoon dried
> Pinch of salt
> 1 quart extra-virgin olive oil

Lightly crush the garlic cloves and put them into a dry 1-quart glass jar along with the ginger and thyme. Pour in the olive oil, then poke a wooden skewer or chopstick down to the bottom of the jar several times to release air bubbles. Follow instructions above for stove-top method. Strain into a clean, dry bottle. You can reserve the garlic and chop it to use immediately in a dish; otherwise, compost the garlic along with the other spent herbs. Refrigerate and use the infused oil within 1 week.

GARLIC

Allium sativum

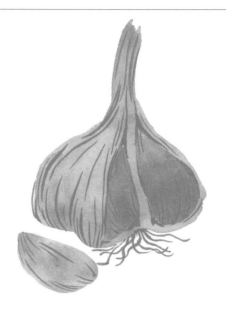

Freshly chopped garlic contains the powerful-smelling allicin, which is partly responsible for garlic's effects against a wide variety of infective agents. Garlic is a renowned antibacterial, antifungal, and antiviral herb, and after centuries of use as a panacea, garlic is now widely used in clinical and pharmaceutical practice to reduce blood pressure and blood cholesterol levels. It's usually regarded as the first protocol for naturally remedying hypercholesterolemia and atherosclerosis. Garlic reduces hyperlipidemia, hypertension, and thrombus formation, making it an ally against thrombosis, or the formation of blood clots in the blood vessels. Garlic has even been shown to be successful in preventing atherosclerosis. It can not only reduce lipid content in the cells of the arteries but also prevent lipid, or fatty cell, accumulation. Of course, garlic bulbs and scapes are most commonly cooked and eaten as food. Many people welcome the addition of garlic in its raw (medicinally active) state to their diet—unfortunately, garlic loses its bactericidal potency and cholesterol-lowering properties when it's cooked.

Mineral-Rich Seaweed Oil for Cooking

 iron-rich | YIELDS 1 QUART

Naturally salty and intense, this oil can be used to deglaze pans, and it makes an excellent cooking oil for vegetables, garlic, onions, and meat. It can also be the base of an intensely delicious pesto or salad dressing that is rich in calcium and iron.

- 3 cups chopped or broken-up dried seaweed, such as arame, dulse, or nori
- 2 cups fresh thyme leaves, or 1 cup dried
- 1 quart extra-virgin olive oil

Put the seaweed and thyme into a 1-quart glass jar. Pour in the olive oil, then poke a wooden skewer or chopstick down to the bottom of the jar to release air bubbles. Follow instructions above for stove-top method. Strain into a clean jar, refrigerate, and use within 1 week.

Light Fennel and Borage Flower Salad Oil

 digestive support | YIELDS 1 QUART

Use this oil as the basis for salad dressings, or drizzle over roasted carrots or fennel bulbs. It's a lovely oil with a light fragrance and the healing benefits of borage, long considered a heart-health herb. The fennel aids in digestion.

    2 cups shredded, packed fresh fennel fronds and/or flowers
    1 cup fennel seeds
    1 cup chopped or shredded, packed fresh borage leaves and/or flowers
    1 quart sunflower or safflower oil

Put the fennel, fennel seeds, and borage into a 1-quart glass jar. Pour in the sunflower oil, then poke a wooden skewer or chopstick down to the bottom of the jar to release air bubbles. Follow instructions above for stove-top method. Strain into a clean jar, refrigerate, and use within 1 week.

Lemony Salad Oil

 refreshing | YIELDS 1 PINT

Give your salads a little zest with an herbal, lemony oil. Add a lemony or wildflower vinegar with salt and pepper to complete a delicious salad.

    1 cup chopped, packed fresh lemon verbena
    1 cup chopped fresh lemon balm
    Zest of 1 lemon (no juice!)
    2 cups sunflower or safflower oil
    Pinch of salt and ground black pepper

Pack the lemon verbena, lemon balm, and lemon zest into a 1-pint glass jar. Pour in the sunflower oil, then poke a wooden skewer or chopstick down to the bottom of the jar to release air bubbles. Follow instructions above for stove-top method. Strain into a clean jar, refrigerate, and use within 1 week.

A-to-Z Warming Oil by Robin Rose Bennett

 immune support | YIELDS 1 QUART

The herbalist Robin Rose Bennett uses this as a culinary oil over sautéed vegetables and also externally, for womb massage and as a topical anti-inflammatory rub for pain. The name may sound like it has every ingredient in the alphabet, but actually it's a combination of just two warming herbs: *Artemisia vulgaris* (mugwort) and *Zingiber officinale* (ginger). These plants soothe and relieve muscle congestion, and they can (but don't necessarily) stimulate delayed menstrual bleeding when used internally as foods and in teas, tinctures, and vinegars. Externally, Robin Rose says the warming, penetrating oil will encourage healthy circulation and ease cramps. "I use it on stiff necks, calf muscles, or anywhere that it might be useful," she says. "A-to-Z Oil helps with sprains, muscle pulls, strains, and inflammation, as well as with menstrual cramps."

Plan ahead to make this recipe: infusing the oil takes several days on a stove top (or several hours in a slow cooker). If you are in a hurry, you can make this oil in a day, but it gets better the longer and more gently it is prepared. It's worth the wait: try serving it over steamed broccoli, steamed asparagus, or roasted potatoes.

1½ cups crumbled dried mugwort leaves and flowers and chopped
   stalks, or 3 cups chopped fresh mugwort (see note)

1 cup grated fresh gingerroot

1 quart extra-virgin olive oil

Put the mugwort and ginger into a small stainless steel pot and cover with the olive oil. Cover the pot and warm it gently over low heat; if it threatens to bubble, turn the heat down or off. Remove the cover to stir it periodically with a wooden spoon. After about 1 hour, remove the pot from the burner. Let it sit, covered, for about 3 hours. Alternatively, you could heat the mixture in a slow cooker on the lowest temperature setting, stirring periodically, for 4 to 6 hours and then let the infused herbs sit for another 24 hours before decanting. (I prefer the stove-top method, but I offer this option because many people love the convenience of the slow cooker.) On the stove top, repeat the warming process once more, being careful not to let the oil bubble. Then, let it sit, covered, overnight.

Repeat the gentle cooking, stirring, and steeping for 2 more days, warming and cooling twice each day. Then strain the oil, squeezing the herbs to extract as much oil as possible. Store in a clean, dry bottle. Shelf life can vary according to conditions; if the oil is kept in a dry place, it can remain good for several years. I have never had this oil turn rancid, but if it does, the flavor and smell would turn unpleasantly sour.

NOTE: Use mature mugwort, in flower if possible.

CLEAVERS
Galium aparine

Lovely cleavers, also spelled *clivers,* grows in tall, gangly bunches that grip onto other vegetation and rock walls and interweave to form mats. Historically, this herb was harvested as a vegetable to be steamed or chopped into soups, but I find it stringy and unpalatable prepared this way. Dried cleavers was used by American colonists to stuff mattresses, giving it the common names "bedstraw" and "ladies' bedstraw."

Cleavers is a renowned herbal remedy employed for "draining" the lymph system, a part of the circulatory system that consists of a network of glands and vessels that shunt lymph fluid directly toward the heart. The lymph system also is made up of lymphocytes—which are produced by the thymus, the bone marrow, and the spleen—and constitutes a part of the immune system as well. Cleavers is believed to help promote proper passage of lymph and interstitial fluid along these vessels and to assist in the removal of foreign bodies and metabolic wastes, especially pathogens. Cleavers is indicated in cases of skin disorders, hepatic dysfunction, urinary dysfunction, cystitis, and prostatitis. Use fresh cleavers only, in teas and infusions or extracted in vinegar.

COMBINING VINEGARS WITH OILS

COMBINE THIS VINEGAR . . .	WITH THIS OIL . . .	TO ACHIEVE THIS FLAVOR:
Strong Garlic Vinegar (page 26)	Strong Garlic Oil (page 36)	Powerful and bold, delicious on robust grilled vegetables
Minty Salad Vinegar (page 28)	Lemony Salad Oil (page 38)	Bright and festive, with high notes of mint and lemon
Green Nettle Vinegar (page 28)	Strong Garlic Oil (page 36)	Nutritious and earthy, a strong foundation for a hearty salad or a dressing for vegetables
Deep-Toning Strengthening Vinegar (with dandelion and ginger) (page 29)	A-to-Z Warming Oil (page 39)	Mildly bitter and warming, best on steamed vegetables and greens
Daily Vinegar (page 29)	Mineral-Rich Seaweed Oil for Cooking (page 37)	Complex and hearty, a mineral-rich dressing for salads
Yang Vinegar (page 30)	Lemony Salad Oil (page 38)	Spicy sage and nasturtium pair with citrusy lemon for salads and fish
Grape Leaf Vinegar (page 32)	Mineral-Rich Seaweed Oil for Cooking (page 37)	Slightly salty, green, and nourishing, great on salads
Vinegar of the Four Thieves (page 33)	A-to-Z Warming Oil (page 39)	Strong and crisp, a standard oil-and-vinegar dressing for salads
Bright Vinegar for Colds (page 34)	Love Your Lymph Oil (page 42)	Strong and crisp, a standard oil-and-vinegar dressing for salads
Fruit Vinegar for Salads (page 34)	Light Fennel & Borage Flower Salad Oil (page 38)	Light and fruity dressing for a light salad of flowers, fruit, and buttery lettuce

Love Your Lymph Oil

 immune support | YIELDS 1 PINT

Use this spicy oil daily if you want to support your immune system. Cleavers is a traditional support herb for the lymph system, a part of both the immune system and the circulatory system.

> 1 cup chopped fresh cleavers
>
> 5 or 6 garlic cloves, peeled
>
> 3 tablespoons chopped fresh parsley
>
> 1 tablespoon chopped fresh horseradish root or prepared horseradish from a jar
>
> 2 cups extra-virgin olive oil

Put the cleavers, garlic, parsley, and horseradish into a 1-pint glass jar. Pour in the olive oil, then poke a wooden skewer or chopstick down to the bottom of the jar to release air bubbles. Follow instructions above for stove-top method. Strain into a clean jar, refrigerate, and use within 1 week.

PESTOS

A well-made basil pesto is a gift from the gods, but don't despair if you don't have sweet or Genovese basil growing in your garden. There are many ways to make a delicious and memorable pesto using the abundant leaves that grow wild all around us—lamb's-quarter, parsley, hyssop, nettle, and dandelion all make spectacular pestos. These pastes taste strong and delightful, and using them as dips for raw carrots or healthy chips is a wonderful way to ingest the vitamins and fiber that are so abundant in our wild foods. Of course, simply stirring pesto into pasta is wonderful, as is using pesto on pizza, flatbreads, and sandwiches.

How to Make Pesto

The traditional way to make a pesto is using a mortar and pestle, which is perfect if you want to make a small bowlful to enjoy immediately. If you'd like to make a larger batch (it freezes so well!), feel free to use a food processor or blender. Nuts, such as pine nuts and walnuts, and sharp cheeses such as Parmesan are typically added to pestos; experiment with your own tastes and adjust these ingredients accordingly. To freeze, scoop the paste into a small freezer container (leaving headroom at the top), drizzle with more olive oil (this prevents contact with air, reducing the risk of freezer burn and discoloration), label, and use within 4 months.

Wild Lamb's-Quarter Pesto
by Robin Rose Bennett

 iron-rich | YIELDS ABOUT 1 CUP

"I'm always making up amounts for my recipes, since I never do anything the same way twice," says the herbalist Robin Rose Bennett. Here she shares a favorite summertime pesto, made all the more special because it starts with a few handfuls of lamb's-quarter leaves harvested under the summer sun. "If your lamb's-quarter is in flower," says Robin, "include the flowers, too, as well as any stalks that are still supple. Experiment with the ratios and measurements—I find it's easiest to blend the solids first with a little oil into a paste, then add more oil until you reach the desired consistency." Use as you would any pesto: on pasta, grains, bread, crackers, or vegetables. This is excellent spread on crudités or dolloped onto tomato, basil, and mozzarella bruschetta.

3 cups lamb's-quarter leaves (and seeds and tender stalks, if desired)

3 or 4 garlic cloves, chopped

¼ cup raw pumpkin seeds (pepitas)

¼ cup sun-dried tomatoes, chopped

½ cup extra-virgin olive oil, plus more if needed

Sea salt, to taste

In a blender or food processor, puree the lamb's-quarters, garlic, pumpkin seeds, and sun-dried tomatoes, stopping to scrape down the sides as needed. While the machine is running, slowly pour in the olive oil until you reach the desired consistency. Taste it, then add salt to your preference. Transfer to an airtight container and drizzle the top with a layer of olive oil to prevent discoloration. Store in the refrigerator for up to 2 weeks.

Spring Weed Pesto by Laurisa Rich

 iron-rich | YIELDS ABOUT 1½ CUPS

My friend and avid gardener Laurisa is very intuitive in the kitchen, throwing together whatever herbs and vegetables she harvested during the day and creating magically tasty meals. She welcomes the volunteer crops of edible and medicinal herbs that sprout up in her ocean-view garden, and she uses them in this pesto to highlight their wild, strong flavors. Gather whatever herbs you have growing, and combine them based on their flavor and scent—let your nose be your guide. If using the miso paste, add less salt.

- ¼ cup raw sunflower seeds
- 1 garlic clove, peeled
- 3 large handfuls of chopped or shredded herbs, such as cilantro, arugula, chickweed, and/or parsley
- 1 teaspoon miso paste, optional
- 1 cup extra-virgin olive oil
- Salt and ground black pepper, to taste

In a blender or food processor, puree the sunflower seeds and garlic into a paste. Pulse in the herbs a little at a time, stopping to scrape down the sides as needed. When pureed, add the miso paste, if using. While the machine is running, slowly pour in the olive oil until you reach the desired consistency. Season with salt and pepper. Transfer to an airtight container and drizzle the top with a layer of olive oil to prevent mold from forming. Store in the refrigerator for up to 2 weeks.

Nettle Dandelion Pesto

 iron-rich | YIELDS ABOUT 2 CUPS

Nettles and dandelion are both prolific, and their fresh, shade-grown leaves can be so succulent that they make an excellent pesto. The flavor is decidedly green, so if you want a little extra scent or spice, add basil leaves. This is a nutritious pesto dip full of minerals as well as many special phytochemicals present in wild plants.

2 cups chopped, packed fresh nettle leaves

2 cups chopped, packed fresh, succulent dandelion leaves (don't use old or wiry leaves)

1 cup chopped, packed basil leaves, optional

2 cups extra-virgin olive oil

1 garlic clove, peeled

½ cup nuts or seeds, such as pine nuts, walnuts, or sunflower seeds

Salt and ground black pepper, to taste

In a blender or food processor, puree the nettles, dandelions, basil (if using), garlic, and nuts, stopping to scrape the sides as needed. While the machine is running, slowly pour in the olive oil. Add the garlic and nuts and puree until desired consistency is reached. Add salt and pepper to taste. Transfer to an airtight container and drizzle the top with a layer of olive oil to prevent mold from forming. Store in the refrigerator for up to 2 weeks.

DANDELION LEAF

Taraxacum officinale

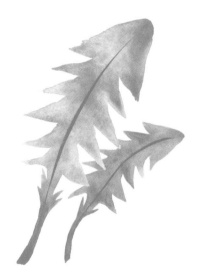

Widely useful for its diuretic effects and to support the liver and digestive system, dandelion leaf directs other herbs toward the urinary tract, helps the body dispel excess water weight, "flushes" the kidneys and bladder, and provides potassium. Because dandelion leaf helps remove excess water from the body, it alleviates the stress on the heart and vascular system caused by excess fluid. Its bitter taste stimulates the secretion of gastric juices and bile, helping the liver and the digestive system, and its diuretic properties make it useful against premenstrual weight gain and bloating. Dandelion leaf can be eaten fresh, juiced, included in tea blends, sautéed and cooked, added to stews and soups, eaten in salads, and included in honeys and syrups.

CHICKWEED

Stellaria media

Chickweed has demonstrable healing effects that are readily evident even to beginners. It demonstrates a very cooling nature that is valuable in hot, inflamed, and infected situations, especially topical ones, and can quickly reduce heat associated with swelling and sepsis, as well as anger. This cooling and lightly sweet-flavored herb is useful in conditions of heat, sluggishness, inflammation, and itching. It's commonly employed as a wash to treat eye infections, as a compress or tincture to reduce fevers, and as a cream or salve to ease itching on the skin due to rashes, heat, sun exposure, or eczema or psoriasis. It is especially cooling and soothing when a compress is made of strong chickweed-leaf tea or pounded fresh chickweed. Look for chickweed beside clear streams or even growing right in the water. Chickweed also grows profusely in rich gardens and can shade new seedlings, but it spreads out in a shrubby fashion from a small central root and can be removed easily. Chickweed is wonderful snipped into fresh salads but does not tolerate cooking; infuse it in honey, vinegar, and oil.

3

HERBAL BUTTERS

Herbal butters add a bit of extra spice, color, and flavor to a dish, and any time you add herbs to food, you're adding extra vitamins and minerals, which is always a good thing.

How to Make an Herbal Butter

There are two methods for making herbal butters: cold and hot. The hot method works well for strong leafy herbs, such as chives or sage, but it is not recommended for delicate flowers, such as violets or calendula. To make butter with these herbs, choose the cold method.

The cold method is the simplest, and it results in a longer shelf life for the butter. This method works best for butter you want to spread on toast or biscuits. Place a stick of butter into a bowl, slice it into 1-inch cubes, and let it soften at room temperature for 10 minutes or so. Mince some fresh herbs, then use a butter knife to smash them into the butter. Once the herbs are evenly distributed, use a rubber spatula to scrape the herbed butter into a storage container with a lid (a small, wide-mouth glass jar works best; avoid narrow openings). Store your herbed butter in the refrigerator. It will offer a pleasantly surprising taste of herbs and will retain its bright yellow color and the vibrant color and freshness of the herbs for 3 to 6 months.

The hot method works best for butter you intend to use for cooking soups, sauces, and stir-fries. Chop the herbs you plan to use and set them aside. Slice the butter into tablespoon-size pieces. A typical ratio is ½ cup chopped herbs to ½ cup butter (1 stick). Heat a saucepan over low heat. Add the butter and chopped herbs and heat very gently, stirring frequently, until you are satisfied with the fragrance of the herbs, about 20 minutes. Be careful not to let the butter burn. This process infuses the flavor and color of the herbs into the butter, and the butter will turn brown (hence the term "brown butter"). Immediately strain the liquid butter into a small jar, or pour the butter, herbs and all, into the jar. If the herbs are included, some will settle to the bottom. Gently shake the jar while the butter is cooling to help distribute the herbs evenly. Store your herbed butter in the refrigerator for 3 to 6 months.

Sage Butter

 immune support | YIELDS ABOUT 1 CUP

Indulge in this aromatic, savory brown butter prepared with the hot method. It's perfect on cheddar biscuits or melted onto butternut squash ravioli or Nettle Ravioli (page 214). My husband likes to use this butter on a special holiday ravioli dish we make with sliced roasted chestnuts and sautéed kale; it also lends its strong antibacterial qualities to a dish of steamed asparagus or a bowl of quinoa or millet.

> 1 cup (2 sticks) salted butter, sliced into tablespoon-size chunks
>
> 4 to 5 tablespoons fresh sage leaves, torn into small pieces
>
> 1 cup sliced roasted chestnuts or walnut halves, optional

Heat a medium saucepan over medium heat. Add the butter and cook until the solids begin to brown. Stir in the sage and chestnuts, if using. Cook until the sage becomes crisp, about 30 more seconds, then immediately pour into a serving bowl. If you will be serving the butter with ravioli, pour the hot butter into a large serving bowl, add the cooked pasta, and toss well. Otherwise, use a spoon to drizzle the hot butter and crisp sage onto steamed vegetables or sautéed fish, or use it as a dip for lobster, mussels, or asparagus. Store any leftovers in the refrigerator and use within 2 weeks.

SAGE

Salvia officinalis

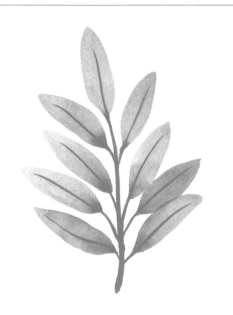

A source of great medicinal, culinary, and even shamanic value in cultures throughout the world, sages are eaten, smoked, inhaled, "smudged," dried, burned, drunk, and tinctured. The astringent common sage treats fever, sore throats, mouth ulcers, and swollen gums, and it helps to dry up mothers' breast milk during weaning. Many menopausal women find the cooling nature of sage helps to relieve hot flashes. Enjoy the astringent and smoky flavor of common sage in butters, vinegars, and honeys.

Garden Butter

YIELDS ABOUT 1 CUP

This creamy butter is thick with flavor and deep in color. Spread it on savory biscuits or scones. You can substitute cream cheese for the butter to make Garden Dip.

- 1 cup (2 sticks) salted butter in 1-inch cubes, at room temperature
- 3 tablespoons minced fresh pungent herbs, such as thyme, oregano, sage, parsley, chives, and/or garlic scapes
- 3 tablespoons minced fresh sweet herbs, such as dill, fennel fronds and flowers, lemon balm, hyssop, and/or basil
- 1 teaspoon grated lemon zest
- ¼ teaspoon salt
- ¼ teaspoon ground black pepper

In a small mixing bowl, mash together the butter and chopped herbs with a wooden spoon or spatula until well combined. Press the mixture into a shallow wide-mouth jar or glass dish. Cap and label the jar, and store in the refrigerator for up to 2 weeks.

Spiced Rose Maple Butter

by Juliet Blankespoor

 stress support | YIELDS ABOUT ¾ CUP

"The synergy of spice and fragrant rose petals infuses rich butter with a sultry flair," says the herbalist and instructor Juliet Blankespoor of this recipe. Enjoy this butter on warm toast, pancakes, waffles, sweet breads, or muffins, and top with fresh berries. Do make sure your rose petals are from plants that haven't been sprayed with chemicals. If you have some maple sugar on hand, you can substitute it for the maple syrup.

- 1 cup (2 sticks) salted butter in 1-inch cubes, at room temperature
- 2 cups loosely packed rose petals
- 1 tablespoon ground cinnamon
- ½ teaspoon ground cardamom
- ¼ cup pure maple syrup
- ½ teaspoon vanilla extract

Put all the ingredients into the bowl of a food processor and blend until smooth. Alternatively, put all the ingredients into a medium bowl and use a wooden spoon to mash them together by hand. Serve immediately. Refrigerate any leftovers and use within 1 week.

Cinnamon Honey Butter

This sweet treat is divine drizzled over freshly baked pretzels, hot from the oven. Sometimes, when our family is making pizza, we save a little dough to make pretzels. Simply roll pizza dough into "snake" shapes, then twist them and bake on a baking sheet or hot pizza stone. As soon as they come out of the oven, pour this butter mixture over them. Cinnamon Honey Butter is a messy, gooey treat that is also delicious on biscuits, scones, or fresh-from-the-oven zucchini bread. Mix up the flavors a little by playing with different infused honeys; for instance, use thyme honey for a bit of pungent flavor or hibiscus honey for a light-pink color and a slightly tart kick.

½ cup (1 stick) salted butter, cut into 1-inch cubes

1 tablespoon raw, unrefined honey

½ teaspoon ground cinnamon

¼ teaspoon ground nutmeg, optional

Pinch of salt

Put all the ingredients into a small saucepan over low heat, and gently warm until the butter is melted. Whisk to evenly incorporate. Immediately drizzle the hot butter on toast, pretzels, or bread. Refrigerate any leftovers and use within 3 days.

4

HONEYS, ELECTUARIES, SYRUPS, AND ELIXIRS

SWEET HONEY IS A NATURAL PAIRING WITH HERBS. There are count-less ways to use honey in the apothecary's kitchen for health, wellness, and vitality. Raw honey contains a bevy of nutrients and enzymes, as well as stored energy, and is more nourishing than commercial or store-bought honey that may have been boiled or adulterated with sugar. Blended with herbs, honey can make a sweet confection or a tart medicine, and even be an ingredient in savory meals. However you prepare it, be sure to keep the heat to a minimum so you don't destroy your honey's beneficial enzymes and vitamins.

The following recipes let honey shine and also bring in other ingredi-ents to make a tasty variety of treats and remedies. Use mild clover honey for a gentle flavor; wildflower honey for a rich flavor; or dark buckwheat honey for a deep, yeasty, and robust flavor and thick consistency. Enjoy making infused honeys, electuaries (pastes of honey with herb powders), syrups (honey with water), and elixirs or oxymels (infused herbal honey with vinegar). Choose tonic herbs that offer their healing energy for what you need most: motherwort and lemon balm for anxiety, blessed thistle and mint for digestive issues, violet and nettle for nutrition. Experiment and let your imagination play, and be sure to do as my eighty-something-year-old friend Ralph does: eat a spoonful of honey every day (and maybe even raise some bees).

HONEYS

When you're new to making foods and drinks using herbs, honeys are a delightful and easy way to start. They're simple to make and convenient to eat, they last a long time without refrigeration, and they're delicious stirred into tea or used in baking. Spend a few minutes in your garden harvesting your favorite aromatic herbs, such as lavender, mint, lemongrass, hyssop, rosemary, or evergreen tips. Chop them coarsely, then indulge: pour honey over them! This is the beginning of a lovely relationship—honey, herbs, and you—and the honey you make will reward you for months to come in breakfasts, snacks, and drinks.

How to Make Infused Herbal Honeys
There are two methods for making infused herbal honeys: hot and cold. Both of these methods produce a tasty and nutritious honey, provided that you use the hot method respectfully and don't overcook the enzymes in the honey.

For the hot method, pour honey into a small saucepan over low heat (not exceeding 110°F), add some chopped fresh herbs, and gently heat the honey until it is translucent. Simply strain the honey into a glass jar and store in a dark place for up to 3 months.

For the cold method, put some chopped fresh herbs into a glass jar and pour room-temperature honey over them. Cover the jar and allow to sit in a cabinet or other cool, dry, dark place for several weeks. Strain into a clean jar, if desired. To strain, slightly heat the mixture (but do not heat it above 110°F) first. Store in a dark place for up to 3 more months.

There is no law that says you have to strain the herbs out of the honey—I have a cold-process honey stored in my pantry in which I infused fresh nettle leaves, and it's delicious to spread the honey and soft leaves together on toast. I also have a jar of cold-process honey with whole thyme sprigs in it, and it's easy enough to spoon out the honey from around the thyme sprigs without having to remove them completely.

If your honey crystallizes in storage, simply place the jar in a saucepan of hot water and heat it through.

Nutritious Nettle Honey

YIELDS ABOUT 1½ CUPS

The combination of nettles and honey is a win-win: it's green, sweet, and full of vitamins. Best of all, it's very easy. Spread this honey on biscuits or stir it into a cup of hot Basic Nettle Infusion (page 95).

2 cups chopped fresh nettle leaves (and tender stalks, if desired)
2 cups light-to-medium raw honey

In a medium saucepan, stir together the nettles and honey. Make sure the nettles are coated well by the honey so none is exposed to air. Cover the pot and allow it to sit on the countertop overnight. In the morning, place the saucepan over very low heat. Gently heat until the honey just liquefies, 2 to 4 minutes. Strain the honey into a labeled jar or crock and store for up to 3 months. The honeyed leaves are good to eat: mix them into oatmeal or spread them on toast.

Citrus Honey

 refreshing | YIELDS ABOUT 1½ CUPS

For those who like a lemony-orange flavor, this sweet treat is rejuvenating and revitalizing. It's also a beautiful golden color and does not need to be strained until you use it, making it a pretty centerpiece on the table in the meantime. Serve this honey over lemon pie or chess pie, or stir it into the Garden Flower Infusion (page 97) or your favorite herbal tea.

½ **cup dried chopped lemon peel**
½ **cup dried chopped orange peel**

½ cup fresh or dried lemongrass ripped into 1- to 2-inch pieces

½ cup fresh or dried lemon verbena leaves ripped into
    1- to 2-inch pieces

2 cups light-to-medium raw honey

1 drop lemon or orange essential oil, optional

Put the lemon peel, orange peel, lemongrass, and lemon verbena into a 1-pint glass jar and pour the honey over them. Using a wooden skewer or chopstick, stir and poke around the herbs to release air bubbles. Make sure the herbs are coated well by the honey so none is exposed to air. Cover the jar and allow to sit for 2 weeks in a dark place. Strain, if desired. To strain, slightly heat the mixture (but do not heat it above 110°F) first. Stir in the lemon or orange oil, if using. To serve unstrained honey, use a small spoon and scoop around the hard pieces, scooping up the soft herbs to eat with the honey. Cap and label the jar and store for up to 3 months.

Deep Forest Honey

 immune support | YIELDS ABOUT 1½ CUPS

This forest-scented honey is lovely in a cup of Earl Grey tea or in a hot cup of tea made from the Lemon Zinger Mulling Blend (page 109). It's also wonderful on biscuits. Ideally, make this in the spring when the hemlocks and spruces are putting out their new bright-green tips.

1 cup new conifer tips, such as hemlock or spruce

½ cup shredded lemongrass leaves

3 or 4 bay leaves

2 cups light-to-medium raw honey

In a medium saucepan, stir together the conifer tips, lemongrass, bay leaves, and honey. Make sure the herbs are coated well by the honey so none is exposed to air. Cover the pot and allow it to sit on the countertop overnight. In the morning, place the saucepan over very low heat. Gently heat until the honey just liquefies, 2 to 4 minutes. Strain the honey into a labeled jar or crock and store for up to 3 months.

CONIFERS

Evergreen trees produce chemical compounds that make them effective medicines. For instance, the delicious new-green tips produced by eastern hemlock (*Tsuga canadensis*) in the spring are rich in vitamin C and have an ascorbic acid flavor; in moderation, these can be eaten raw for a quick snack in the woods, or they can be steeped in boiled water for a very fragrant and strong-tasting tea. The sharp balsamic and woody fragrance of spruces (*Picea* spp.) and Scotch pine (*Pinus sylvestrus*) indicates the presence of essential oils pinene, limonene, cineole, camphene, and borneol—making their needles excellent additions to steam baths, poultices, compresses, and oils. In the kitchen, use evergreen tips and leaves in syrups and honeys, and don't forget to put a little in your wildflower vinegars for an extra kick.

BORAGE
Borago officinalis

Long ago, borage was used in drinks for courage, well-being, vigor, and stamina. It was widely believed to confer these traits and was the principal ingredient in the cordial. Although its edible leaves are cooling and cucumber-scented, it used to be considered warming. We now know its leaves are high in potassium salts, which may be partly responsible for its invigorating and mild energy-giving effects. Today many herbalists use borage to support the nervous system. Try using fresh borage leaves and flowers in ice cubes and cold drinks, in salads, and in vinegars, honeys, elixirs, syrups, and hot herbal milks.

Stress-Relief Honey

 stress support | YIELDS ABOUT 1½ CUPS

Eat or drink a small amount of this honey daily to support your body and mind through stressful times; these herbs are traditionally used to help ease stress and to reduce anxiety. Borage is historically known as the herb that "gives courage," and tulsi, or holy basil, is renowned for its lovely flavor and its calm, centering energy. This honey is delicious and doubly effective stirred into Gratitude Tea (page 86) or Heart-to-Heart Tea (page 91). Other herbs that would work nicely in this blend are rhodiola root, Saint-John's-wort flower, and red clover blossom.

1 cup fresh borage flowers and leaves, or ⅓ cup dried

½ cup dried holy basil (tulsi) leaves

2 tablespoons dried chopped ashwagandha root

2 cups light-to-medium raw honey

In a medium saucepan, stir together the borage, holy basil, ashwagandha, and honey. Make sure the herbs are coated well by the honey so none is exposed to air. Cover the pot and allow it to sit on the countertop overnight. In the morning, place the saucepan over very low heat. Gently heat until the honey just liquefies, 2 to 4 minutes. Strain the honey into a labeled jar or crock and store for up to 3 months.

Spring Tonic Honey by Jan Berry

 nourishing | YIELDS 1 CUP

The farm hobbyist and herbal blogger Jan Berry spreads this spring tonic honey over hot buttered biscuits or toast and adds it to her tea. You can strain out the flowers from the infused honey, or "alternatively, you can do what I do, and just leave the flowers in and spoon around them," she says. "You can actually eat the honeyed flowers by the spoonful, too. I find them quite yummy!" She suggests taking 1 tablespoon of this infused honey per day to help alleviate seasonal allergies. It can even be used as a face wash for acne and dry skin: gently pat it on, then rinse with warm water.

Small handful of fresh dandelion flowers

Small handful of fresh violet flowers

1 cup raw honey

Remove the green stem and fringes (sepals) from the dandelion flowers and keep the heads of yellow petals. Remove the stems from the violet flowers. Stuff the flowers into a ½-pint glass jar and pour the honey over them. Using a wooden skewer or chopstick, stir and poke around the herbs to release air bubbles. Make sure the herbs are coated well by the honey so none is exposed to air. Cover the jar and allow to sit in a dark place for up to 2 weeks. Strain, if desired. To strain, slightly heat the mixture (but do not heat it above 110°F) first. Cap and label the jar and store for up to 3 months.

Angelica Honey for Digestion

 digestive support | YIELDS ABOUT 1½ CUPS

I love angelica. In my garden it is often covered with bees and wasps, who seem to adore its fragrance. This lovely herb smells heavenly and is traditionally used as a carminative—an herb that helps ease indigestion. This is a great honey to stir into a cup of after-dinner herbal tea (such as Daily Respite Tea, page 87, or Nice Nerves Tea, page 91), and is especially useful after a heavy meal. To harvest angelica seeds, snip off the entire cluster, or umbel, when the seeds are dark, full, and ripe-to-almost-dry. Use them fresh in this recipe, or dry them on a screen or newspaper and store in a jar in a dark pantry for later use in tea blends or butter. Use whatever fresh herbs and seeds from the list are available.

> 1 cup chopped mixed fresh herbs—choose from the following:
>> Angelica leaves or stems (wilted 20 minutes on newspaper)
>> Catnip leaves
>> Hyssop leaves
>> Lemon balm leaves
>> Bee balm leaves
>> Fennel leaves and/or flowers
>> Dill leaves and/or flowers
> 1 tablespoon crushed fennel seeds
> 1 tablespoon crushed angelica seeds
> 2 cups light-to-medium raw honey

In a medium saucepan, stir together the mixed herbs, fennel seeds, angelica seeds, and honey. Make sure the herbs are coated well by the honey so none is exposed to air. Cover the pot and allow it to sit on the countertop overnight. In the morning, place the saucepan over very low heat. Gently heat until the honey just liquefies, 2 to 4 minutes. Strain the honey into a labeled jar or crock and store for up to 3 months.

ANGELICA

Angelica archangelica and *A. sinensis*

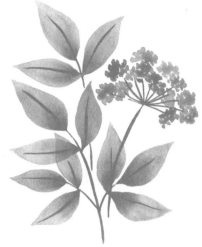

The many species of fragrant angelica have long been used for healing digestive upset, gas, bloating, and external conditions of ringworm and itching. The aromatic and flavorful roots and stems have been candied and the seeds chewed for their flavor and to dispel flatulence. *Angelica sinensis*, also called dong quai, dang qi, or Chinese angelica, is a favorite among midwives for its antispasmodic effect on the uterus. Dong quai is often used to treat dysmenorrhea (painful menses), pelvic congestion, endometriosis, and fibroids, especially because of its antispasmodic effect on smooth muscle. Experiment with its bright, pungent flavor, which is somewhere between mint and licorice: use it in teas, syrups, honeys, candies, and electuaries.

CATNIP

Nepeta cataria

This lovely gray-green plant in the mint family spreads easily and reseeds itself throughout the garden. Gather the silvery stalks and strip off the leaves and tiny flowers to dry them. They emit an enchanting dusky mint scent that is sedative and calming to humans, unlike its effect on cats, which are well known to be stimulated by it. A tea made from catnip is mild and soothing, with a full-bodied mouthfeel, and when mixed with a bit of honey it is a wonderful warm tea to give children before bed. Mildly sedative, catnip helps ease children's bedtime nervousness, insomnia, and night fears. Let the children help you collect it and make the tea. Catnip is carminative, providing mintlike treatment for gas, bloating, and indigestion. Excellent in tea blends, it's also great in honeys, elixirs, pestos, and stews.

An electuary is simply honey with powdered herbs mixed into it. The result is a thick paste that can be spread on toast or savored by the ½ teaspoon. It can also be diluted in a cup of hot tea, adding a thickness and flavor to the tea that can be wonderful in the depths of winter. This is a good way to make use of bitter herbs because their taste is masked in the sweet depths of the honey; ground ginger and motherwort and goldenseal powders are great in electuaries because they can taste too strong on their own. Any herb powder can be used: my friend Missy's four-year-old daughter, Violet, has decided (and rightfully so) that her favorite electuary is honey mixed with cocoa powder.

Electuaries tend to get thicker as they age, so don't be surprised when you open your jar and discover it has hardened somewhat. Keep this in mind when making your electuary; consider adding less powder for a thinner consistency than your ideal, to compensate for its getting thicker over time. Also, feel free to experiment with colors: adding hibiscus powder to your honey will create a bright crimson electuary; adding nettle or lemongrass powder will make it green; goldenseal creates a dark gold, orange-brown electuary. Store your electuary in a shallow wide-mouthed jar or small crock rather than a tall, narrow jar; it will be much easier to get to. Stored in a dark, cool pantry or cabinet, the electuary will last more than a year.

ECHINACEA
Echinacea angustifolia, *E. purpurea,* and *E. pallida*

Echinacea, or purple coneflower, has experienced a great amount of scientific and clinical research. The glycoside-rich root is a proven antimicrobial and antiviral and has shown laboratory activity against *Streptococcus* bacteria and also *Staphylococcus aureus* infection. Echinacea is effectively used for many illnesses where bacterial, viral, parasitic, or fungal infection is present. It aggressively stimulates the body's defense system, activates macrophage activity to combat tumor cells, and increases white blood cell count and activity. Although fresh and tinctured echinacea tastes strong and tingly on the tongue, the dried chopped root or powder is milder; use fresh or dried echinacea in tea blends, decoctions, and mulling spices, and use the powder form in smoothies and electuaries. Avoid echinacea if you have hayfever, are pregnant, or have an immune disorder.

Tangy Electuary for Immune Support

 immune support | YIELDS ABOUT 1 PINT

A tangy-tasting boost of immune system support is always welcome in the winter. Echinacea is hailed as an immune-support herb thanks to its polysaccharides, among other chemicals. Ascorbic acid powder is easy to purchase at a health food store; it makes the honey tangy, tart, and sometimes a bit granular. Rose hips are naturally high in vitamin C, and thyme is renowned as an immune-support herb. All these herbs are easy to find as powders, but you can also grind them yourself in a coffee grinder.

 2 cups light-to-medium raw honey

 1 to 2 teaspoons echinacea root powder

 1 to 2 teaspoons rose hip powder

 1 to 2 teaspoons hibiscus powder

 1 to 2 teaspoons dried thyme leaves

 1 to 2 teaspoons ascorbic acid (vitamin C) powder

Pour the honey into a shallow wide-mouth jar. Add 1 teaspoon each of the echinacea root powder, rose hip powder, hibiscus powder, thyme, and ascorbic acid and stir with a wooden skewer. Add more of the herb powders, thyme, and ascorbic acid until you achieve a consistency a little runnier than you want (it will thicken with time). Cap and label the jar and store in a cabinet or other dark place.

Spicy Ginger Electuary

 immune support | YIELDS ABOUT 1 CUP

This is one of the easiest electuaries to make, because most of us have a little ground ginger in our baking cupboard. Ground ginger, or ginger powder, is a highly fragrant spice with a strong flavor that pairs well with cinnamon and nutmeg. This spicy electuary can be thinned and spread on toast or biscuits, or nibbled from the edge of a spoon when you're feeling under the weather and need a pick-me-up.

 1 cup raw honey

 2 to 4 teaspoons ground ginger

 1 teaspoon ground cinnamon

Pour the honey into a shallow wide-mouth jar. Add 2 teaspoons of the ginger and the cinnamon and stir with a wooden skewer. Add more ginger until you achieve a consistency a little runnier than you want (it will thicken with time). Cap and label the jar and store in a cabinet or other dark place.

Cinnamon Molasses Spread for Toast and Biscuits

YIELDS ABOUT 1 CUP

This spicy spread is divine on biscuits. It's unusual to mix molasses into a honey electuary, but the effect is like a cozy winter morning in Grandma's kitchen.

1 cup raw honey

1 to 2 teaspoons ground cinnamon

1 to 2 teaspoons ground cardamom

1 to 2 teaspoons ground allspice

¼ to ½ teaspoon ground ginger

2 tablespoons molasses

Pour the honey into a shallow wide-mouth jar. Add 1 teaspoon each of cinnamon, cardamom, and allspice, ¼ teaspoon ginger, and the molasses and stir with a wooden skewer. Add more of the ground spices until you achieve a consistency a little runnier than you want (it will thicken with time). Cap and label the jar and store in a cabinet or other dark place for up to 1 month (the shelf life of this electuary is reduced due to the molasses).

SYRUPS

Syrups are great fun to make and easy to use; they can be drizzled on pastries or stirred into hot teas. They can be light and delicate or robust and rich. Herbal syrups contain all the benefits of the herb in a sweet, liquid form, making them a useful method for giving children medicines that would otherwise taste too bitter or strong, such as motherwort, garlic, or horseradish. Syrups can be combined with vinegar for making elixirs (see page 72), used as part of a cordial or liqueur recipe, or blended with a cordial to pour over ice cream as a treat. Because sugar is the base, syrups should be indulged in only occasionally. Syrups differ from infused honey and electuaries in one important regard: because water has been added,

CINNAMON

Cinnamomum spp.

Long valued for its heavenly scent and used as an incense with aphrodisiac properties, cinnamon was one of humanity's earliest commodities. It was one of the exotic spices responsible for the Eastern spice trade, and it is mentioned numerous times in the Bible, as well as in Chinese herbals as early as 2700 BCE.

Medicinally, cinnamon is aromatic, pungent, fragrant, carminative, and astringent, and it is used as a glandular system stimulant and a stomach antacid. I use it alongside elder and thyme for colds and flu. As a carminative, cinnamon's aromatic oils help stimulate proper digestive function, ease bloating, dispel gas, and promote gastric integrity. Its warming qualities indicate its application in cases of fever as well as in Ayurvedic formulas for those with sluggish or "kapha" dispositions. Use cinnamon in limited quantities, because its component coumarin is toxic to the liver and kidneys in moderate-to-high concentrations.

It's easy to make electuaries with ground cinnamon and honey and to include cinnamon bark in teas and oils. Use tiny amounts in herb powder blends, smoothie blends, hot herbal milks, puddings, and even stews.

their shelf life is much shorter (generally only a few days), and they must be stored in the refrigerator.

The formation of a little mold on the surface of the syrup is not uncommon, especially if you choose not to add brandy. If you see mold on the surface, simply remove it with a spoon and transfer the syrup to a clean jar. However, if you see mold deeper in the syrup, throw it out and start a fresh batch.

How to Make a Syrup

There are three basic ways to make a syrup:

TEA FIRST, LIGHT SYRUP. Make a strong herbal tea, strain it into a glass jar, and add enough honey or sugar to make a syrup to your desired consistency.

TEA FIRST, HEAVY SYRUP. Make a strong herbal tea, strain it into a small saucepan, and add sugar. Bring the mixture to a boil, then lower the heat and simmer, stirring frequently, until the sugar dissolves and the syrup reaches your desired consistency.

HONEY FIRST, LIGHT SYRUP. Infuse your honey with herbs or dried fruit (using the method in "How to Make Infused Herbal Honeys," page 53), strain it into a glass jar, and whisk in enough water or tea to create your desired consistency.

Regardless of the method you choose, be sure to refrigerate your syrup immediately, and use it within a few days. Also consider adding brandy, which will extend its life a few more days.

A note about sugar: most recipes in this book avoid sugar. Many syrup recipes call for a certain amount of herbs boiled in water and then double that amount of sugar, which is too much sugar, in my opinion—the herbal goodness gets lost. For these syrups, try to use as little sugar and honey as possible to achieve the consistency and flavor you desire.

Nourishing Soul Syrup with Oats and Linden
by Suzanna Stone

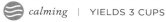 *calming* | YIELDS 3 CUPS

Put linden, oats, and roses together, and you have a sublime blend for supporting a frazzled nervous system—all three herbs are considered nervous system tonics. Linden is also a traditional cardiovascular tonic, and rose is a tonic of the emotional "heart." Suzanna Stone, herbalist and director of Owlcraft Healing Ways school in central Virginia, uses these healing herbs together as a delicious syrup and says it is grounding, nourishing, and relaxing to those who suffer from nervous exhaustion. "It is one of my favorite sweet medicines," she says, "to help heal a wounded spirit, and to open and help heal a grieving heart." As a tonic, adults should take 1 to 2 tablespoons daily, and children under 12 should take 2 teaspoons once or twice a day.

6 cups water

1 cup dried milky oats

½ cup dried rose petals

½ cup shredded dried linden leaves and flowers

5 cardamom pods

1 cup local honey

2 tablespoons 80-proof brandy

LINDEN

Tilia europaea, T. americana, and *T. cordata*

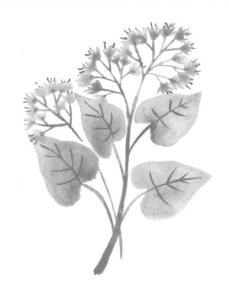

Lindens are lovely tall trees with large heart-shaped leaves and "dripping" flowers that can be harvested in a cluster. When dried, the flavonoid-rich flowers are sweet smelling and sticky and difficult to separate. The leaves and flowers are cardiotonic, which means they are strengthening to the cardiovascular system and will reduce blood pressure even though they do not contain cardiac glycosides (if they did, they would be called cardioactive herbs). As a tonic for long-term and sustained care, not acute conditions, linden is used to support blood vessel integrity and normalize heart muscle contractions. Linden is commonly used in respiratory illnesses, especially to soothe dry, unproductive, hacking coughs. The flowers are traditionally used to ease anxiety and relieve nervous tension, making linden flower a beloved nervine tonic, while the leaves are used to reduce mild fevers. Brew linden in teas and infusions, and include it in honeys, syrups, vinegars, and powder blends.

In a large saucepan over high heat, combine the water, oats, rose petals, linden, and cardamom and bring to a boil. Reduce the heat to medium-low and simmer until the liquid is reduced by half, about 20 to 30 minutes. You should have 3 cups of liquid. Strain into a glass jar, add the honey, and stir until the honey is dissolved. Stir in the brandy as a preservative and cap and label the jar. Kept refrigerated, this syrup will last 4 to 6 weeks.

Summertime Strawberry-Mint Syrup by Blaire Edwards

 refreshing | YIELDS 1 PINT

"This is a syrup I love to make in the summertime," says herbalist Blaire Edwards, "when strawberries are cheap and my mint plant is growing like the precious weed that it is." This is a fruity and refreshing syrup that's wonderful drizzled over fruit tarts or mixed with infused vodkas for a potent drink. For a refreshing pick-me-up beverage, Blaire suggests mixing ½ cup of this syrup with 2 cups watermelon juice and 1 cup seltzer water and serving over ice.

> 5 cups fresh strawberries
>
> 1½ cups water
>
> 1 cup sugar
>
> 4 to 5 tablespoons chopped fresh mint leaves

In a large saucepan over high heat, combine the strawberries, water, and sugar. Bring to a boil, then reduce the heat to low, cover, and simmer for 10 minutes. Strain the mixture, pressing the strawberries to get all the juice. Return the strained liquid to the saucepan and place over high heat. Bring to a boil again and add the mint. Reduce the heat and simmer, uncovered, until it is thick and syrupy, 5 to 10 minutes. Pour into a glass jar, cap, and label. Store in the refrigerator for up to 3 days.

Respiratory Syrup

 immune support | YIELDS ABOUT 1 PINT

These herbs are helpful for soothing a hacking cough, easing inflamed lungs, and calming a throat made raw during a cold or the flu. Take by the ½ teaspoon as needed.

> 2 cups water
>
> 2 teaspoons shredded dried mullein leaf
>
> 2 teaspoons chopped dried elecampane root
>
> 1 teaspoon chopped dried licorice root
>
> 1 cup raw honey

In a small saucepan over high heat, combine the water, mullein, elecampane, and licorice. Bring to a boil, then reduce the heat and simmer, uncovered, until the liquid is reduced by half, about 10 minutes. Strain the liquid into a medium bowl and allow to cool. Once cool, whisk in the honey. Pour the syrup into a glass jar, cap, and label. Store in the refrigerator and use within 3 days.

ELECAMPANE

Inula helenium

This is a lovely and stately biennial herb, growing very tall and producing profuse dark green leaves and a few large, bright yellow flowers. The root is very useful for a persistent, hacking cough and for bronchitis; elecampane is my first choice when someone can't sleep due to coughing. It's gentle enough for children and is an ideal bronchial antispasmodic, helping to keep coughing at bay long enough for a good night's sleep. Steep fresh elecampane in vinegar or white wine, or enjoy it in tea or a decoction. Elecampane makes an excellent honey or syrup.

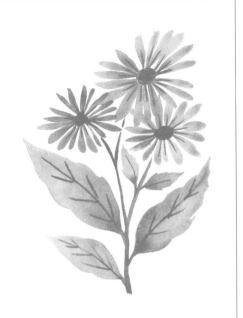

Iron Anemia Syrup

 iron-rich | YIELDS ABOUT 1 PINT

Wild dandelion and nettles are renowned for their mineral content, especially iron, and yellow dock reportedly helps the body assimilate iron. According to a publication by the North American Institute of Medical Herbalism, burdock, catnip, chickweed, horsetail, marshmallow, and red raspberry are also very high in iron. In this syrup, we combine high-iron herbs with high-iron foods, including molasses, to make a syrup that can be enjoyed by the teaspoon when your energy is down or when you're feeling depleted.

2 cups water

2 tablespoons dried chopped dandelion root, or
   ¼ cup plus 2 tablespoons chopped fresh

2 tablespoons dried chopped yellow dock root or burdock root, or
   ¼ cup plus 2 tablespoons chopped fresh

2 tablespoons shredded raspberry leaves

5 or 6 sprigs of fresh chickweed (omit if the fresh herb is not available)

2 tablespoons crumbled dried nettle leaves, or
   ¼ cup plus 2 tablespoons chopped fresh

10 raisins

2 dates

½ cup raw honey

½ cup molasses

In a small saucepan over high heat, combine the water, dandelion, yellow dock, raspberry, chickweed, nettles, raisins, and dates. Bring to a boil, then reduce the heat and simmer, uncovered, until the liquid is reduced by half, about 10 minutes. Strain the liquid into a medium bowl and allow to cool. Once cool, whisk in some of the honey and molasses, taste, and add more as needed to reach the desired sweetness. Pour the syrup into a glass jar, cap, and label. Store in the refrigerator and use within 3 days.

Bitters Syrup

 digestive support | YIELDS ABOUT 1 PINT

Bitters have been used in digestive tonics for centuries, often consumed as a tiny aperitif before a meal. Bitter herbs stimulate digestive juices and prepare our bodies for food. These bitter herbs pair well with honey to create a remedy that is both pleasant and effective. Don't make this syrup too sweet; instead, let the bitterness shine through. This is not a tonic, but it is an effective remedy to take in small amounts before meals to improve digestion.

2 cups water

2 tablespoons chopped dried rue leaves

2 tablespoons chopped dried motherwort leaves

2 teaspoons chopped dried blessed thistle leaves

1 teaspoon caraway seeds

1 cup raw honey

In a small saucepan over high heat, combine the water, rue, motherwort, blessed thistle, and caraway seeds. Bring to a boil, then reduce the heat and simmer, uncovered, until the liquid is reduced by half, about 10 minutes. Strain the liquid into a medium bowl and allow to cool. Once cool, whisk in the honey. Pour the syrup into a glass jar, cap, and label. Store in the refrigerator and use within 3 days.

YELLOW DOCK
Rumex crispus

Common in poor soils and throughout the garden, yellow dock (also called granny dock and curly dock) sports an edible yellowish-brown root high in bio-available iron. It can be used in an iron-rich syrup for anemic women and those needing extra iron, such as after surgery. The greasy leaves can be eaten when very young and tender (1 to 2 inches long) and are good lightly steamed and sprinkled with vinegar. The roots can be chopped and included in stir-fries. The seeds are often pounded and included in recipes for dyeing fabric or wool. Sometimes yellow dock is included in formulas for lymph system drainage because of its alterative effect, even though it provides no direct immune system support. It works very well in apple cider vinegar.

RASPBERRY
Rubus idaeus

Raspberry canes are bluish-purple, and raspberry leaves are soft green above and silver underneath. People eat the berries of the second-year canes, and the fresh leaves of the first-year canes make a nourishing tea cherished by midwives for toning the uterus. Traditionally considered a uterine tonic, Western herbalists encourage pregnant women to drink several calcium-rich cups a day to strengthen the uterus and build strong bones. Often used as an astringent douche for leukor-rhea, or inflammation of the cervix, a water infusion of raspberry leaves and roots makes a useful, drinkable astringent remedy for dysentery and diarrhea yet is mild enough for children. Use raspberry leaf in honeys, syrups, elixirs, tea blends, and vinegars.

Antioxidant Berry Syrup by Brittany Nickerson

 heart support | YIELDS ABOUT 1½ CUPS

The herbalist Brittany Nickerson's tasty syrup features autumn-ripened fruits that are rich in antioxidants and bioflavonoids. "These are plant-based constituents that support the cardiovascular system and immune system," says Brittany, "and they reduce the harmful effects of stress on the body. Hawthorn berries and rose hips both ripen in the fall after warm days and cool nights have sweetened them up—they have a sweet and slightly sour flavor that makes a delicious syrup for adults and children alike." Brittany suggests using this syrup as a flavoring with water, sparkling water, or tea or as an addition to fruit and vegetable juices. Try it in salad dressings, stir-fries, baking, or as a topping on desserts.

2 cups filtered or well water

¼ cup fresh hawthorn berries, or 2 tablespoons dried

¼ cup fresh rose hips, or 2 tablespoons dried

2 tablespoons chopped fresh orange peel, or 1 tablespoon dried

½ cup raw honey

¼ cup brandy, optional

In a small saucepan over high heat, combine the water, hawthorn berries, rose hips, and orange peel. Bring to a boil, then reduce the heat to medium-low and simmer, uncovered, until the liquid is reduced by half, about 10 minutes. Strain the liquid into a medium bowl and stir in the honey, then transfer to a glass jar. Alternatively, strain directly into a jar, add the honey, and shake to combine. Allow to cool, then stir in the brandy, if using. Cap and store in the refrigerator for 4 to 6 weeks. (The brandy is an optional preservative; it will help your syrup last 2 to 3 months in the refrigerator.)

Lymph Tonic Syrup

 immune support | YIELDS ABOUT 1 PINT

Cleavers is traditionally used to support the lymph system, which is part of both the immune and circulatory systems. Use fresh cleavers, not dried, and chop it up fine (or even pound it into a paste in a mortar and pestle) before adding to the honey. This syrup combines cleaver tea with cleaver honey to make a lovely lymph-supporting syrup.

2 cups packed fresh cleavers (stalk and leaves)

1 cup raw honey

2 cups water

Pound 1 cup of the cleavers into a paste with a mortar and pestle, or pulse in a food processor. Chop the remaining 1 cup of cleavers. In a small saucepan, combine the pounded cleavers with the honey. Here you have two options: either gently heat the pan over low heat until the honey is liquefied, or cover the pan and let it sit on the countertop overnight. After the honey is liquefied or after steeping overnight, strain into a medium bowl.

Meanwhile, in another small saucepan over high heat, combine the chopped cleavers with the water. When the mixture approaches boiling,

MOTHERWORT

Leonurus cardiaca

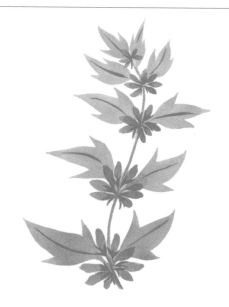

One of my favorite herbs, motherwort was affectionately named *Leonurus cardiaca* because it gives the strength of "the heart of a lion." It is commonly called motherwort because it is the *wort,* or herb, of the mother, especially the exhausted mother of young children, and it is often tinctured and taken to relieve anxiety, nervous tension, exhaustion, and fear and is especially useful for cases where fear leads to heart palpitations, irregular heartbeat, and hypertension. These self-sowing seed heads produce tiny sharp spines, so wear gloves while harvesting it. Long revered in the folk traditions of Russia and Europe, motherwort strengthens heart tone, and it is a nervine tonic used to soothe jangled nerves and even hysteria. Its bitter principle makes it a useful digestive aid. Use motherwort for congestion in both the pelvic region and the cardiac region, and to ease nervous tension without sedation. It's too bitter for drinking in a tea; instead, prepare motherwort in syrups, vinegar-and-honey elixirs (oxymels), and vinegars.

ROSE HIPS

Rosa spp., especially *Rosa rugosa*

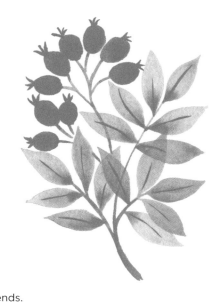

Rose hips, the astringent fruits that appear after the rose has shed its bloom, are very high in vitamin C. A syrup made from the hips can be used all winter as a preventive. The pleasantly tart taste mixes well with elderberries and ginger to create a potent syrup used equally well as a pancake syrup and a cough medicine. Another favorite way to enjoy rose hips is to create an elixir from the chopped hips brewed with apple cider vinegar and honey. This infused vinegar can be taken straight or used as the base for salad dressings. Rose hip powder adds a tart flavor to smoothies and spice blends. Whole rose hips can be added to mulling blends.

reduce the heat to medium low and simmer until the liquid is reduced by about half, about 10 minutes. You should have about 1 cup of liquid. Allow the tea to cool to room temperature and strain.

Pour the cooled tea into the bowl with the infused honey a little at a time, whisking to combine. Add tea until the syrup is your desired consistency. Pour the syrup into a glass jar, cap, and label. Store in the refrigerator for 3 to 4 days.

ELIXIRS

An elixir is a divinely inspired combination of something sweet—such as honey or sugar—and something sour, such as vinegar or lemon juice. It's enough to make the mouth pucker, but instead of a harsh bite it packs a lovely sweet-tart punch.

Elixirs, also called oxymels, can be very valuable medicinally. Often when we have a cold or the flu, we want to take very strong herbs such as ginger, garlic, goldenseal, motherwort, or rose hips. Sometimes these taste too strong or bitter to get down pleasantly—hence, an oxymel. It's another delicious way to take what might otherwise be nasty medicines. And as tonic and fortifying remedies, elixirs can be taken daily.

How to Make an Elixir

There are two basic ways to make an elixir:

VINEGAR FIRST. Infuse the vinegar with the herbs or fruits of your choice, then strain the vinegar and add honey.

HONEY FIRST. Infuse the honey with the herbs or fruits of your choice, then strain the honey and add vinegar.

Either way, you're creating a blend of roughly half vinegar and half honey, but the proportions are completely open to interpretation and experimentation. Taste as you go; it's easy to add a bit more sweetness or a little more acidity. Feel free to substitute lemon juice for the vinegar, but recognize that the shelf life may be shorter.

Store your elixir in a small bottle in the refrigerator and use within a few weeks. Take it by the spoonful when you're feeling the need, or add some to a cup of hot tea for a sweet-tart pick-me-up.

BLESSED THISTLE

Cnicus benedictus

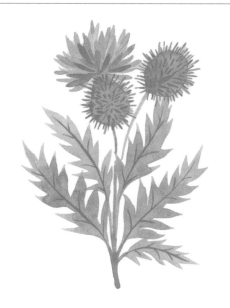

Folk medicine gives contradictory information about the historic uses of blessed thistle. Also called Our Lady's milk thistle and holy thistle, this plant is often confused with milk thistle, *Silybum marianum,* but they are not related. Blessed thistle was reputed to be helpful during the European plagues of the Middle Ages, when it was used as a vulnerary, or wound healer. The leaves are very bitter, and these bitter qualities may help ease digestion, another use for which it is well known. It is considered by folk herbalists to be a mild galactagogue—that is, to promote milk production—though the herbalist Aviva Romm declares it is not as potent as fenugreek, caraway, dill, or fennel. Use the extremely bitter leaves of blessed thistle in tiny amounts in elixirs, syrups, and honeys.

Respiratory Support Oxymel by Suzanna Stone

 immune support | YIELDS ABOUT 2 CUPS

This tasty remedy makes taking medicine easy. Herbalist Suzanna Stone blends these healing herbs with sweet and sour flavors to create a traditional elixir that children will love. "I love oxymels, with their blend of the sweet with the sour," says Suzanna. "This recipe is perfect for getting you through cold season and helps move congestion out of the body easily." Take it by the spoonful, or stir into a bit of water or tea. Adults should take 1 tablespoon one to four times daily, and children under 12 should take 2 to 3 teaspoons three times daily.

- **4 cups apple cider vinegar**
- **1 yellow onion with skin, coarsely chopped**
- **5 garlic cloves, coarsely chopped**
- **1 tablespoon fresh rosemary leaves, or 1 to 2 teaspoons dried**

1 tablespoon chopped fresh hyssop leaves, or 1 to 2 teaspoons dried

1 tablespoon fresh thyme leaves, or 1 to 2 teaspoons dried

¼ cup crumbled dried mullein leaf

2 cups local honey

In a medium saucepan over high heat, combine the vinegar, onion, garlic, rosemary, hyssop, thyme, and mullein and bring to a boil. Reduce the heat and simmer, uncovered, until the volume is reduced by half, about 20 to 30 minutes, or up to an hour for a very concentrated oxymel. You should have about 2 cups. Strain, and return the infused vinegar to the saucepan and place over low heat. Stir in the honey and heat until it dissolves. Pour into a glass jar, cap, and label. Store in the refrigerator for up to 6 months.

MULLEIN

Verbascum thapsus and *V. densiflorum*

One of the easiest to identify of the wildflowers, mullein is a soft-leaved fuzzy friend to children and hikers alike. The plant originated in the arid Mediterranean, and its soft leaves gave it the nicknames velvet dock and flannelwort. A biennial, the herb produces leaves in a rosette the first year, and the second year it sends up a towering stalk on which its yellow flowers blossom. Early Europeans used a warm compress of the leaves on "piles" or hemorrhoids and external wounds such as burns and tissue tears. They also asserted that witches and evil spirits could be kept away by the light of a flaming mullein-stalk torch. When colonists introduced mullein to the New World, native peoples soon learned its value and used the leaves as an ingredient in their *kinnick-kinnick*, a smoking mixture used for both ceremony and lung health. The tincture and tisane are also used internally as a pulmonary tonic and aid for dry, hacking coughs. Include mullein leaf and flower in your teas, syrups, honeys, and oils.

Triple Berry Oxymel by Heather Thurber

The herbalist and Ayurvedic massage practitioner Heather Thurber shares the history of her favorite family recipe, delicious Triple Berry Oxymel:

> Some of my earliest and best memories are summers spent with my Gram at her farm in Hodgeman County, Kansas. Combining herbs, honey, and fruit from the farm with wild-crafted indigenous plants, Gram was always concocting syrups, vinegars, and "health tonics," as she called them. She was very well known for her Triple Berry Oxymel. She would often make big batches, and we would drive it around the countryside delivering it to other farm families and members of Gram's church community.
>
> To make her Triple Berry Oxymel, Gram would always make a big batch of homemade Granny Smith apple cider vinegar, which would then be infused with wild-harvested blackberries, huckleberries, and red raspberries. This infusion was then combined with raw honey and a spearmint leaf infusion. The combination was then cured for several weeks in a cool, dark cabinet and later decanted. The Triple Berry Oxymel was one of the most delicious syrups and would be used as medicine for upper respiratory ailments or put on salads or enjoyed in sparkling water with ice. Today I make the same traditional oxymel and enjoy it for health and wellness throughout the year.

Made in a three-step process, this elixir requires some prep time—a few weeks—so plan accordingly. Once the vinegar, honey, and mint infusions are prepared, all three are combined to create a delicious and nutritious remedy.

FOR THE INFUSED VINEGAR

- 2 cups apple cider vinegar
- ½ cup blackberries
- ½ cup red raspberries

2 cups raw honey

1 cup dried blueberries

FOR THE WATER INFUSION

2 cups chopped fresh spearmint leaves, or 1 cup shredded dried

3 cups water

To make the infused vinegar, combine the ingredients in a large glass bowl and cover it with a lid or cloth. Let it sit for 2 weeks, unrefrigerated, in a cupboard or dark pantry. Stir it once a day. After 14 days, strain out the berries and set the infused vinegar aside.

To make the infused honey, combine the ingredients in a large glass jar, cover, and let sit for 2 weeks, unrefrigerated, in a cupboard or dark pantry. Shake the jar vigorously twice a day. After 14 days, strain out the berries and set the infused honey aside.

To make the water infusion, combine the mint and water in a medium saucepan over low heat. Heat for 20 to 30 minutes or until the infusion is dark and fragrant. Strain out the mint leaves and set the infusion aside.

To prepare the elixir, combine the infused vinegar, honey, and water in a large saucepan over very low heat. Heat until the honey dissolves, about 5 minutes, whisking gently. Pour the mixture into a glass bowl and allow it to cool. Decant the elixir into sterilized bottles with screw-on lids. Store the bottles in a cool, dark place or in the refrigerator for up to 2 months.

Champagne Grape Elixir

by Robin Rose Bennett

 heart support | YIELDS 1 QUART

For a fun way to take your grape medicine, here is an elixir the herbalist Robin Rose Bennett says she made as an experiment that turned out to taste divine. "It's fantastic for your circulation, and it tastes absurdly good," she says. Drizzle it over biscuits, pound cake, or ice cream; or blend with Robin's Grape Leaf Vinegar (page 32) to make a refreshing salad dressing.

1 cup fresh champagne (Corinth) grapes or your favorite
    red or purple grapes

1 cup 100-proof vodka

2 cups wildflower honey

In a wide-mouth 1-quart glass jar, gently mash the grapes. Pour in the honey and vodka and stir. Adjusting the proportions to suit your taste, fill the jar to a ¼ inch of the top, then cap and label it. Store in a cool, dry place for 6 weeks, then decant into smaller glass jars or bottles.

Vitality Elixir

 stress support | YIELDS ABOUT 1 PINT

I had the good fortune to contribute to the musician Sally Taylor's fantastic artistic experiment called *Consenses*. She curates projects in which one person creates a piece of art (such as a song, a dance, or a painting), and Sally sends this artwork to another artist, who interprets it in his or her own medium. For instance, she sent me an evocative photograph of a lovely woman reclining in the sunshine, and I interpreted that photo in my own medium: as a tea blend. Sally then sent my tea to be brewed and enjoyed by another artist, who interpreted the tea in a video, and then another artist interpreted that video as a dance performance. I found these "chains" fascinating to explore when her production premiered on Martha's Vineyard, and I think they attest to the vivid imagination of artists and the inherent collective symbolism in art.

This elixir is based on the tea blend I made for Sally, which was a simple yet evocative blend of cardamom, lemon verbena, and vanilla. Here, it is combined with lemongrass, honey, and a bit of apple cider vinegar to give it a sweet-tart kick with hints of softness and spiciness. It makes an arousing and delicious syrup to drizzle over vanilla ice cream or sip off the spoon.

> ¾ **cup shredded dried lemon verbena, or 2 cups chopped fresh**
> ½ **cup dried chopped lemongrass, or 1 cup chopped fresh**
> ¼ **cup cardamom seeds or crushed pods and seeds**
> **1 cup raw honey**
> **1 teaspoon vanilla extract**
> ½ **to ¾ cup apple cider vinegar**

In a small saucepan, combine the lemon verbena, lemongrass, and cardamom, and pour the honey over them. Stir well to make sure all the herbs are coated in the honey. Cover the saucepan and let sit on the countertop overnight. In the morning, place the saucepan over very low heat and heat just until the honey liquefies, about 5 minutes, being careful not to overheat it. Carefully strain the infused honey into a bowl. (Either compost the herbs or remove the cardamom pods and spread them on toast.)

Stir in the vanilla extract. Add ½ cup of the vinegar first, then add more, 1 tablespoon at a time. Add enough vinegar to give the elixir a sweet-and-sour tang that is enjoyable to sip by the spoonful. Pour into a 1-pint glass jar. Cap, label, and store in the refrigerator for up to 3 weeks.

LEMONGRASS

Cymbopogon spp.

Native to India and Southeast Asia, this thickly growing grass produces a lovely lemon flavor and has been cultivated for culinary use for centuries. Used as a tea and in soups, curries, and citrus desserts, it is also a valuable insect repellent when used externally in sprays or soaps. Snip bits of fresh lemongrass into soups, use it dried in tea blends, and use both fresh and dried liberally in honeys, syrups, and mild-flavored vinegars.

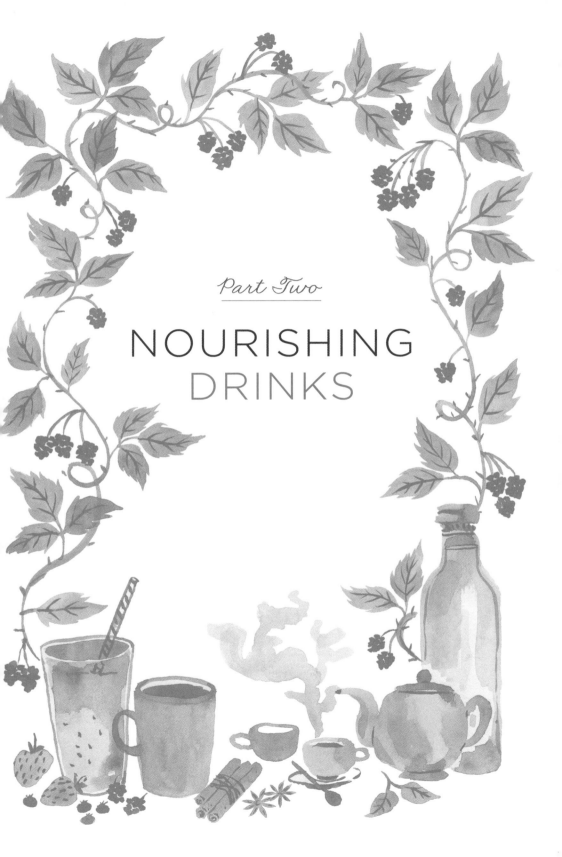

Part Two

NOURISHING
DRINKS

5

HERBAL TEAS, INFUSIONS, AND DECOCTIONS

AHH, TEAS! Herbal teas are the heart and soul of herbal medicine making. I have a cupboard brimming with jars and bags of delightful dried-herb concoctions that are ready to brew, and I love to blend new tastes together and experiment with flavors. It's relatively inexpensive to try making blends—buying herbs in the bulk section of a health food store allows you to get as little or as much as you want, and only a small handful of fresh herbs from the garden will dry into enough to make at least a dozen cups of tea. And because you need only 1 teaspoon of dried herbs per cup of boiling water, it's quick and cheap to blend a few different herbs together, brew it for a few minutes, and taste. With scores of tasty and fragrant herbs available for making delicious drinks, it's easy to experiment and explore until you find a handful of herbs or tea blends that suit your taste and life-style. Keep a glass canning jar of your favorite dried-herb tea blend on an easy-to-reach shelf in your healing kitchen, and reach for it often.

While many people enjoy herbal teas (officially *tisanes*, as true "tea" comes only from a *Camellia* plant) for their flavor alone, others recognize that sipping a few cups of lemon balm tea can calm the nerves, and a couple of cups of ginger tea can relieve an upset stomach. Lots of herbs are good at relieving symptoms, but I especially appreciate those helpful herbs that strengthen and nourish preventively. These herbs—such as rhodiola, nettle, alfalfa, oatstraw, dandelion, mint, and holy basil (tulsi)—are among the best herbs to use daily in teas, syrups, powder blends, and foods. These are the nutritious herbs, which contain a surprising amount of iron, potassium, magnesium, and loads of vitamins. Steeping them in hot water releases these compounds into your cup so you can enjoy the benefits of their taste and nutrition all at once.

Making herbal teas is so easy—it requires very little in the way of equipment and doesn't take much time. The most enjoyable part is collecting the fresh herbs, but even if you purchase dried herbs, you still get to enjoy the sensory experience of handling them, blending their colors and textures, and of course inhaling their aroma. Steeping herbal teas takes only 5 to 15 minutes, depending on the herb. Crafting a ritual around your tea-brewing experience will help you ease stress and create something dependable and enjoyable—a ritual to look forward to each morning, afternoon, or evening. Let it help you relax and escape. Or let it rejuvenate you: the abundant healing herbs contain a multitude of compounds that can either ease anxiety or stimulate the mind, whichever you choose, and most of them contain the vitamins and minerals you need to stay strong and feel refreshed.

Each of the following recipes has been created to brew a quart of tea—four cups, which is the generally recommended daily amount to drink for optimum benefit. If you want less, simply reduce the amount of dried tea you include: 1 teaspoon of dried herbs per 1 cup of boiling water. When using fresh herbs, think "handful" per cup, or 1 tablespoon of chopped fresh herbs, which will generally fit in the palm of your hand.

HERBAL TEAS

True "tea" is made from the *Camellia sinensis* plant, a lovely shrub grown primarily in China whose leaves contain caffeine. This shrub is the source of all true teas, including black, green, pu-erh, and oolong, in which the leaves are dried or fermented. Herbal teas are made from any other herb and generally contain no caffeine, and they are more accurately called tisanes.

When leaves, flowers, and soft plant parts are steeped in water for several hours or overnight (much longer than a tea) and then strained, the resulting beverage is called an *infusion*, and when seeds, roots, twigs, and harder plant parts have been simmered in water and strained, this makes what is called a *decoction*. (See page 92 for more on infusions and decoctions.) Many of these recipes could also be made into infusions—allowing the herbs to steep much longer in the water; however, I generally don't brew mints this way. Peppermint, spearmint, hyssop, and bee balm—all these wonderful minty flavors—seem better when they are brewed for a shorter period of time, as a tisane. But feel free to experiment with length of brew time and combinations to find the tastes that suit you.

Herbal teas have a lot to recommend them, and you can do much more with them than just drink them. Turn your freshly brewed herbal tea into a base for a honey syrup (see page 62), a lotion base, a hair rinse, a compress for a sore joint, a foot soak, an addition to your bath, and much more. Here, we'll simply enjoy herbal teas as divinely inspired beverages that build our bones, hair, skin, teeth, and nails; restore our vitality with vitamins and trace minerals; ease digestion; soothe us at nighttime or refresh us in the morning; and that nourish us during times of illness with hot, fruity, or deeply satisfying flavors.

How to Make Herbal Tea

To make a general herbal tea, or tisane, brew 1 teaspoon of crumbled dried herbs in 1 cup of just-boiled water. Steep the herbs in the water for about 8 minutes or according to the directions in the recipe. Strain the tea into a Thermos or a jar and store it in the fridge, for up to 2 days, to be reheated as desired.

Iced Flower Berry Zinger

 refreshing | YIELDS 1 QUART

Enjoy this fruity, colorful tea as a hot beverage in the winter or iced in the summer. Its ginger and elderberry make it a potent immune-support beverage, and the hibiscus makes it a mild heart tonic also. To make a pitcher of iced tea, brew it hot, then chill it and serve with slices of fresh lemon and orange.

1 tablespoon dried chopped gingerroot, or ½ cup chopped fresh
1 tablespoon dried elderberries

Herbal Teas, Infusions, and Decoctions

2 teaspoons dried hibiscus flowers

Honey, to taste

½ teaspoon ascorbic acid (vitamin C) powder, optional

Combine the ginger, elderberries, and hibiscus in a 1-quart glass jar. Pour enough boiling water over them to fill the jar. Tightly cover and let steep for 8 to 10 minutes, according to your taste. Strain, and sweeten with honey to taste. Stir in the ascorbic acid, if using. Store the hot tea in a Thermos, or refrigerate in a pitcher or glass jar for iced tea. Drink 2 to 4 cups throughout the day.

Nerve Tonic Tea

 stress support | YIELDS 1 QUART

Mix these herbs together and store the blend in a tin so it's available whenever you're ready to make this delicious tea. This is a superb digestive blend and also a lovely nighttime tea because it helps the body relax and soothes the nerves. This is an excellent blend for those who are so anxious or stressed it affects their digestion or their sleep.

1 tablespoon dried chopped gingerroot

1 tablespoon dried chamomile flowers

2 teaspoons crumbled dried spearmint leaves

1 teaspoon fennel seeds or crumbled dried fennel leaves

1 teaspoon dried lavender flowers

½ teaspoon crumbled dried stevia leaves

Combine the ginger, chamomile, spearmint, fennel, lavender, and stevia in a 1-quart glass jar. Pour enough boiling water over them to fill the jar. Tightly cover and let steep for 8 to 12 minutes, according to your taste. Note that the stevia will develop a slightly saccharine flavor if allowed to steep for too long. Strain the hot tea into a Thermos, and drink 1 to 2 cups when feeling stressed, as a digestive aid, or before bed. Store any remaining tea in a glass jar in the refrigerator, to reheat as desired.

CHAMOMILE

Matricaria recutita

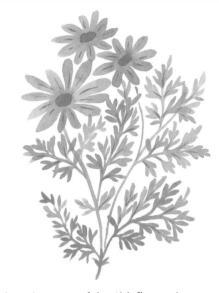

Chamomile is a time-honored traditional remedy and one of the most popular herbal remedies ever used. It is valued throughout Europe and the United States for a variety of hot, irritated, and inflamed conditions. Soothing chamomile infusion is calming for infants, children, and adults and is especially helpful for an infant's cranky condition due to colic, indigestion, burping, or hiccups. Chamomile is also used in acute conditions of panic, distress, nervous exhaustion, and fear, as well as chronic anxiety and chronic indigestion. Its blue essential oil, azulene, is a powerful anti-inflammatory and antimicrobial agent. Mildly bitter, chamomile has long been used to ease menstrual cramps and treat digestive spasms. Use it especially in tea blends, as well as in syrups, honeys, electuaries, powder blends, and smoothies.

HIBISCUS

Hibiscus rosa-sinensis

In the Western herbal tradition, hibiscus is considered cooling, demulcent, and tonic, and it is often used as a nervine tonic. Alternatively, in Ayurveda hibiscus is indicated as an emmenagogue to stimulate menstrual flow and as a contraceptive, uses for which it is being studied in India today. High in antioxidants, hibiscus flowers' pleasantly tart taste makes a lovely addition to teas and infusions, and they impart a bright pink color when brewed. Include hibiscus freely in teas, infusions, syrups, electuaries, and smoothie blends.

HOLY BASIL (TULSI)

Ocimum tenuiflorum and *O. gratissimum*

The pleasant, mild basil-like fragrance of this herb makes it a truly wonderful tea; it has a smooth mouthfeel and a light flavor that combines well with other herbs, such as ashwagandha and rose, but it is equally good by itself. Also called tulsi or tulasi, holy basil is a "Rasayana" herb in Ayurvedic medicine, meaning it supports rejuvenation and the building up of strength, especially after an illness or incident. Current research is showing it is also an immune supporter and may be useful in asthma and inflammatory allergic responses. Enjoy holy basil in teas, infusions, syrups, puddings (use a tulsi tea as the base in Rose Petal Rice Pudding, page 221), and it is excellent in honey.

Gratitude Tea

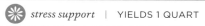 *stress support* | YIELDS 1 QUART

I've come to love this simple blend, as it has a pungent aroma mildly reminiscent of garden basil but is also very light and flowery, with an exotic flavor so prized in tulsi, also called tulasi or holy basil. The roses give it a sweet airy quality so that altogether this is a very soothing and refreshing tea, particularly wonderful for easing stress or when you feel you need to take a deep breath.

> 4 to 6 teaspoons dried holy basil
>
> 2 teaspoons crumbled dried rose petals (red or pink)
>
> Honey, to taste, optional

Combine the holy basil and rose petals in a 1-quart glass jar. Pour enough boiling water over them to fill the jar. Tightly cover and let steep for 8 to 12 minutes, according to your taste. Strain the hot tea into a Thermos and sweeten with honey to taste, if desired. Drink 2 to 4 cups throughout the day.

Mental Clari-Tea

 clarity & memory | YIELDS 1 QUART

This is a lemony-minty blend meant to open up the blood flow to the brain and increase cognitive function. Lemon balm is traditionally used to improve concentration and strengthen memory and is beloved by herbalists for supporting those with ADD/ADHD in their efforts to concentrate and focus. Mixed with hyssop leaf (a bright, minty-flavored herb) and mint (which is refreshing and revitalizing), lemon balm is right at home. This is a wonderful morning pick-me-up tea that can be enjoyed hot or iced.

> 2 teaspoons crumbled dried hyssop leaf
>
> 2 teaspoons crumbled dried lemon balm leaf
>
> 2 teaspoons crumbled dried mint (any kind)
>
> Honey, to taste, optional

Combine the hyssop, lemon balm, and mint in a 1-quart glass jar. Pour enough boiling water over them to fill the jar. Tightly cover and let steep for 8 to 12 minutes, according to your taste. Strain the hot tea into a Thermos and sweeten with honey to taste, if desired. Drink 2 to 4 cups throughout the day.

Daily Respite Tea

 stress support | YIELDS 1 QUART

Use this tea for a light pick-me-up during the day or as a calming blend at night. Nettle doesn't give its full force in this light green tea; instead, it offers its mellow flavor alongside oatstraw, which is light and pleasant. Ashwagandha is also light and rather bland, while rhodiola brings the whole blend together with a warming tart punch. This isn't a zinger; instead, it is a pleasant tea that takes away the pangs of hunger, eases stress, and lends a feeling of satisfaction and fulfillment. (If rhodiola is unavailable, use holy basil.)

 1 tablespoon crumbled dried nettle leaves

 1 tablespoon crumbled dried oatstraw or dried milky oats

 2 teaspoons dried chopped ashwagandha root

 1 teaspoon dried chopped rhodiola root, or 2 teaspoons crumbled dried holy basil leaves

 Honey, to taste, optional

Combine the nettles, oatstraw, ashwagandha, and rhodiola in a 1-quart glass jar. Pour enough boiling water over them to fill the jar. Tightly cover and let steep for 8 to 10 minutes, according to your taste. Strain the hot tea into a Thermos and sweeten with honey to taste, if desired. Drink 2 cups when feeling stressed or at bedtime. Store any remaining tea in a glass jar in the refrigerator, to reheat as desired.

Minty Delight Tea

 digestive support | YIELDS 1 QUART

For those who love a good, strong mint tea, this is high on the list of wonderful blends. Get the zing you want from the mint, add a little sweet minty hyssop, and top it off (like a high note in perfumery) with lemon verbena. It's very soothing when hot, and delicious and sparkly when chilled.

 3 to 4 teaspoons crumbled dried peppermint or spearmint leaves

 1 tablespoon crumbled dried hyssop leaves

2 teaspoons crumbled dried lemon verbena leaves

Honey, to taste, optional

Combine the mint, hyssop, and lemon verbena in a 1-quart glass jar. Pour enough boiling water over them to fill the jar. Tightly cover and let steep for 8 to 10 minutes, according to your taste. Strain, and sweeten with honey to taste, if desired. Store the hot tea in a Thermos, or refrigerate in a pitcher or jar for iced tea. Drink 2 to 4 cups throughout the day.

Summary Solstice Tea

 refreshing | YIELDS 1 QUART

Celebrate the longest day of the year with traditional solstice herbs, enjoyed for their sacred presence in gardens and along the roadsides at this pivotal point in the year. Offering a variety of colors and flavors, these herbs are plentiful in midsummer, giving us reason to harvest them and give thanks for their abundance. Play around with the amounts, using less or more depending on what grows near you. Do use fresh herbs in this recipe, to take advantage of the lively energy of the solstice.

Bring the flavors of the various herbs together with a bright burst of orange: steep orange slices in the tea itself, use orange slices to decorate a pitcher of iced tea, or squeeze orange juice into the tea when you're ready to drink it.

3 tablespoons fresh Saint-John's-wort leaves and flowers

3 tablespoons chopped fresh bee balm leaves and petals

3 tablespoons lavender leaves and flowers

3 tablespoons shredded red clover blossoms

Handful of other edible herbs of choice, such as nasturtium, catnip, mint, and/or calendula

Honey, to taste

1 orange, sliced, or the juice from 1 orange

Combine the Saint-John's-wort, bee balm, lavender, red clover, and other herbs in a 1-quart glass jar. Pour enough boiling water over them to fill the jar. Tightly cover and let steep for 10 to 15 minutes, according to your taste. Strain, and sweeten with honey to taste, if desired. Add the orange slices or juice to the hot tea and store in a Thermos, or refrigerate in a pitcher or glass jar and add the orange slices before drinking it iced. Drink freely throughout the day.

OATSTRAW

Avena sativa

This grass has been grown for millennia in the Mediterranean and Near East as a nourishing food and medicine. Valued for their smooth and creamy mucilage, oat plants offer us green milky tips, stalks (oatstraw), and fruit (oats and groats). The grains can be cooked as a breakfast cereal, and the oatstraw can be brewed into a tea. Oatstraw is occasionally used in tincture form.

The straw and grain are extraordinarily nutritious, high in calcium, iron, phosphorous, magnesium, and the B vitamins. Herbalists employ oats and oatstraw to restore bone and muscle mass, strengthen capillaries, lower cholesterol levels, and nourish hormonal systems. Both oats and oatstraw are nervine tonics, supporting the nervous system and alleviating stress, and herbalists recommend consuming cooked oats and oatstraw teas during pregnancy and breast-feeding. Use fresh milky oat tops (that is, the immature seeds) and dried oatstraw, with their bland and unassuming taste, in honeys, herb powder blends, and smoothies.

RHODIOLA

Rhodiola rosea

A mild cardiotonic and rejuvenator, rhodiola root is considered to have a cooling effect, making it ideal for those with anxiety, stress, or overwork that causes elevated heart rate, high blood pressure, ulcers, and exhaustion. Its use is established in the herbal traditions of Scandinavia, Eastern Europe, and especially Russia, where the root is used to improve mental clarity and support the heart and lungs. Use it in teas, vinegars, honeys, elixirs, and smoothies.

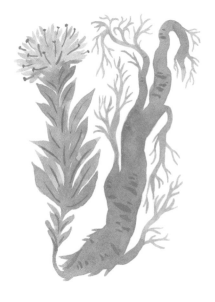

SPEARMINT AND PEPPERMINT

Mentha spicata and *M. piperita*

Full of volatile, or essential, oils, all the members of the mint family aid in digestive function, reduce gas, and reduce symptoms associated with ulcers. I generally use peppermint to enhance circulation, to induce sweating (or alternatively, to cool down a hot person), to support mental clarity and blood flow to the brain, and externally to stimulate blood flow to an area and fight infection. I use peppermint's milder and sweeter cousin spearmint for children and the infirm, as it has many of peppermint's stimulating and digestive properties but without the punch and the heat. Spearmint supports other herbs as a "vehicle" or "dispersant" in formulas, such as herbal combinations for coughs, bronchitis, pelvic inflammation, asthma, colds, influenza (though peppermint is more effective here), and for young women suffering uterine pain and cramping with menarche. Both of these mints are delicious as teas, but they can quickly overwhelm in an infusion. Use them in blends with a variety of herbs, keeping in mind peppermint yields a stronger, sharper flavor while spearmint is a little sweeter. They make an outstanding infused honey and are useful in elixirs, vinegars, oils, rice and grain dishes, chai blends, and herb powder blends.

SAINT-JOHN'S-WORT

Hypericum perforatum

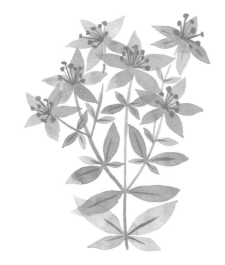

A lovely wildflower, oil-rich Saint-John's-wort has been found to be clinically effective in those with anxiety, improving their ability to sleep, to relax, and to cope with daily stress, and it may be valuable for those with posttraumatic stress disorder. For depression that is mild to moderate, Saint-John's-wort has routinely proven more effective than a placebo and just as effective as tricyclic antidepressants, without the common side effects of prescription medications. Because of its possible contraindications with a long list of prescription medications (such as some anticoagulants and other antidepressants), care must be taken when using Saint-John's-wort extracts long-term. Saint-John's-wort makes a lovely tea and infuses well in vinegar.

Nice Nerves Tea

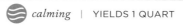 *calming* | YIELDS 1 QUART

For those days when you need a little soothing help from a nice cup of hot tea, this blend will become your go-to. It's soothing, relaxing, and wonderful for giving you the sense of "*ahhh.*" Blend the herbs together and store them in a favorite tin or clear glass jar, and scoop a few teaspoons for your bedtime tea ritual.

> 3 to 4 teaspoons dried chamomile flowers
>
> 3 to 4 teaspoons crumbled dried holy basil leaves
>
> 1 teaspoon crumbled dried rose petals (red or pink)
>
> Honey, to taste, if desired

Combine the chamomile, holy basil, and rose petals in a 1-quart glass jar. Pour enough boiling water over them to fill the jar. Tightly cover and let steep for 8 to 12 minutes, according to your taste. Strain, and sweeten with honey to taste, if desired. Store the hot tea in a Thermos, or refrigerate in a pitcher or glass jar for iced tea. Drink 2 cups when feeling stressed or at bedtime. Store any remaining tea in a glass jar in the refrigerator, to reheat as desired.

Heart-to-Heart Tea

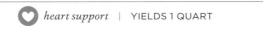 *heart support* | YIELDS 1 QUART

I remember coming upon a grove of hawthorn trees in the mountains of western North Carolina and being amazed at the length of the spiny thorns—some more than 2 inches long. In fact, the hawthorn is a prize. It looks daunting, but the leaves, twigs, and berries of this tree are a true delight. They brew into a very tasty, naturally sweet tea that is renowned as a mild heart tonic, helping to lower high blood pressure. Many herbalists like to use it to support not only the physical heart muscle but also the ethereal heart—the emotions—especially for those facing trying circumstances, grief, loss, or heartache.

Taste this brewed tea before adding sweetener—you may find it's sweet enough on its own.

> 1 tablespoon plus 1 teaspoon crumbled
>   dried hawthorn leaves

Herbal Teas, Infusions, and Decoctions

1 teaspoon whole dried hawthorn berries

1 teaspoon crumbled dried rose petals

Combine the hawthorn leaves and berries and rose petals in a 1-quart glass jar. Pour enough boiling water over them to fill the jar. Tightly cover and let steep for 10 to 15 minutes, according to your taste. Strain, and sweeten with honey to taste, if desired. Store the hot tea in a Thermos, or refrigerate in a pitcher or glass jar for iced tea. Drink 2 to 4 cups throughout the day.

Women's Tonic Tea

 stress support | YIELDS 1 QUART

A hormone-balancing tea for women of all ages, this peace-bringing blend is deliciously strong. Crush the berries and seeds with a mortar and pestle if you want an even stronger flavor.

2 teaspoons dried chaste-tree berries

1 teaspoon dried angelica seeds or chopped stems or root

1 teaspoon fennel seeds

1 teaspoon dried hibiscus flowers

Combine the chaste-tree berries, angelica, fennel, and hibiscus in a 1-quart glass jar. Pour enough boiling water over them to fill the jar. Tightly cover and let steep for 10 to 15 minutes, according to your taste. Strain, and sweeten to taste, if desired. Store the hot tea in a Thermos, or refrigerate in a pitcher or glass jar for iced tea. Drink 2 to 4 cups throughout the day.

INFUSIONS AND DECOCTIONS

Infusions and decoctions are a bit more substantial than teas, or tisanes. *Infusions* (a term used by herbalist Susun Weed) and *standard brews* (a term used by herbalist Juliette de Bairacli Levy) refer to the product of dried leaves, flowers, and other aerial parts of an herb having been steeped in initially boiling water for a long time, at least 4 hours and often overnight, and then strained out. This allows time for the minerals and chemical compounds to extract into the water and results in a robust beverage—richer in nutrients, stronger in flavor, with a much thicker mouthfeel and a darker color than a tisane. This drink is full of beneficial plant compounds:

BEE BALM

Monarda fistulosa and *M. didyma*

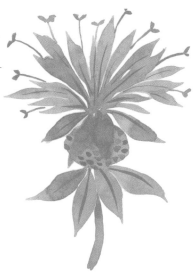

I saw my first patch of bee balm at the Old Homeplace farmstead in the rich valley of Sugar Grove, North Carolina, when I lived there in the 1990s. The owner, then in his eighties, had planted little patches of this wildflower decades before, and they had grown and spread so that, coming over a hill or around a curve along the steep driveway up the mountain, you would see bright red-capped clusters of tall, stately flowers. These often grew taller than me, and I was somewhat disappointed the first year I planted scarlet bee balm (*M. didyma*) in my garden on Martha's Vineyard to discover they only grew to about two feet high. However, by the second and third years they were shoulder- and head-high, and I've also discovered since then varieties of *M. fistulosa* with violet, blue, and orange-red flowers. The species can be used interchangeably.

Also called Oswego tea and bergamot, bee balm leaves offer a strong, minty scent and flavor. I don't find the flowers to be as flavorful as the leaves, but they are beautiful in honey and vinegar. The Tewa Indians reportedly ate the boiled leaves with meat, and many native nations ate the herb boiled or used in external poultices to relieve symptoms of colds, fever, flu, pain, headache, and congestion. I've found the best way to use bee balm is in teas, infusions, honeys, vinegars, syrups, and smoothies. Experiment with their bright, minty flavor in stews and soups, and use the blossoms for a punch of color in ice cubes and sprinkled fresh on salads.

vitamins, minerals, anthocyanidins, antioxidants, phenols, and more. And if you're using the right herbs, it's a fantastic tonic as well.

Decoctions are at least as substantial as infusions but are brewed from the harder parts of the plant: the seeds, bark, and roots. The brewing time is a bit longer, and the pot actually simmers for some time on the stove top, covered, to more fully extract all the herbal goodness. After simmering, the pot often remains covered with the herbs steeping inside for an hour or more to create a strong, rich beverage. Decoctions usually taste richer and bolder, and are sometimes more bitter, than infusions.

How to Make an Infusion

Brew your infusions using a lot of herbs—often herbalists use 1 ounce of dried herbs to 1 quart of boiling water, but 5 to 6 teaspoons per quart usually will suffice and yield a satisfying and mineral-rich brew. Minerals require time to extract into the water—more than the 5 to 12 minutes typical for brewing most teas. Plan to begin brewing your infusion in the evening, so you can cover it and let it steep overnight, and then strain in the morning. Or begin brewing in the morning and let it sit throughout the day for an evening treat. To drink your infusion, strain it and reheat if desired. Add honey or a bit of stevia if it needs some sweetness. Often, it doesn't!

Feel free to substitute herbs that grow near you or ones that are blooming at the moment, and dry them in a shady, well-ventilated area such as the top of the stairs or on a shady porch. You can make all these recipes with fresh herbs, too, but remember to use three times the quantity. For example, you would use 1 teaspoon of dried nettle leaves for a cup of tea, or 3 teaspoons (1 tablespoon) of fresh nettle leaves. Also keep in mind that some herbs have bitter glycosides and can become unpleasant when they're brewed too long; for example, an infusion that contains dandelion leaves, motherwort, or chamomile may be pleasant after 5 minutes but unbearably bitter after 15.

How to Make a Decoction

Similar to an infusion, a decoction is made from the harder or woodier parts of the plant; these parts generally need more nudging to release their healing properties into the water. Plan on 1 to 2 teaspoons of chopped root, bark, or seeds per cup of water. Combine the herbal material and cold water in a saucepan and bring to a boil. Cover with a lid, reduce the heat, and simmer for 20 minutes. For an extra-strong brew, remove the pan from the heat and allow it to sit, covered, for an additional 10 to 20 minutes. The resulting "tea" will be strongly aromatic and strongly flavored. Licorice root can be steeped along with the other herbs to add sweetness, if desired. If you'd like to include the softer parts of herbs (such as leaves or flowers) in the blend, add them during the last 5 to 8 minutes of simmering or steeping. Strain and drink.

Basic Nettle Infusion

 iron-rich

In the summer one of my favorite things to do is to brew a large pot of rich, dark-green nettle infusion from the fresh leaves and stems of stinging nettle. I use our deep pasta pot and make a little more than a gallon at a time. My whole family loves it, and we drink it quickly: I'll put the whole gallon in the refrigerator for iced tea on hot days. When I drink it, I feel invigorated and fortified. It's a very strengthening tea, and in the winter I miss it. Using dried herbs, however, gives a very close approximation, and this nutritious brew is invaluable in the depths of the winter months.

Here are three ways to make a very satisfying, nutrient-rich, healing, vibrant, delicious pot of tea using *Urtica dioica*—nettle, one of my favorite plants. Experiment to find your favorite method.

FRESH IN THE POT
YIELDS ABOUT 1 GALLON

This is the ideal way to enjoy all that nettles have to offer. It produces a deep-green, mineral-rich infusion that is heavier than a tea, with a fairly thick mouthfeel. It's substantial. It's a meal in a cup.

Get out your tongs and gloves and harvest entire stalks of nettle, cutting them a few inches from the ground. This is best to do in the spring, from the time the nettles are about 6 inches high until they are full-grown and about 4 feet high. The stalks can be harvested later, when they are in bloom or seed, but I think nettles are tastiest before the plant has flowered. (To bloom, a plant pulls its energy from the leaves and puts it into developing the flowers; for this tea, however, we want the freshest, most succulent leaves.)

Collect all the stalks in a large paper grocery bag. For a large pot of infusion, collect fifteen to twenty 6- to 8-inch stalks.

Bring a large pot of water to a boil. Using tongs, pull a nettle stalk from the bag and hold it upside down over the pot. Using scissors, snip each leaf off the stalk and let it fall into the water. Note: if you plan to reuse the strained-out nettles later in the Nettle Dandelion Pesto (page 44), Nettle Cream Cheese Dip (page 168), or another goodie, snip only the leaves (not the stalk) into the water. If you plan on composting everything, you can also snip the stalk into the water along with the leaves.

When all the leaves from all the stalks have been snipped into the pot, use your scissors to cut them up a bit in the pot, randomly chopping to slice them into smaller pieces. Turn off the heat and cover the pot. Allow the pot to sit undisturbed for the next 4 to 8 hours. Strain, and sweeten if desired, setting aside the used nettle leaves for another optional use. Drink the infusion freely. Refrigerate any leftovers and drink within 1 day.

DRIED IN THE POT
YIELDS 1 TO 2 QUARTS

Get the same goodness year-round by using dried nettles. It's a much less intensive process than using the fresh herb and yields a tasty, strong cup of nettle infusion with all the same minerals and all that chlorophyll.

Place 1 to 2 packed cups of dried nettle leaves in a large saucepan. Pour 1 to 2 quarts of boiling water over them. Cover the pan and allow it to sit undisturbed for the next 4 to 8 hours. Strain, and sweeten if desired. Drink the infusion freely. Refrigerate any leftovers and drink within 1 day.

DRIED IN THE PERCOLATOR
YIELDS ABOUT 1 QUART

This is a lovely method for creating a strong healing drink on a cold winter day. I like to use my grandmother's old ceramic percolator with its glass top and place it on our woodstove. The brew gets stronger the longer it percolates, but be careful not to forget about it or all the water may evaporate out.

Fill the percolator with fresh cold water. Place 1 cup of crumbled, packed dried nettle leaves in the percolator's filter basket.

Place the percolator on a woodstove or over medium-low heat on the stove top. With either heat source, bring the water to a boil, let the percolator do its job for roughly 20 minutes, and then remove it from heat. An electric percolator may be used if it can be set to percolate up to 20 minutes.

Strain. Sweeten with honey and/or add milk, if desired. Refrigerate any leftover nettle infusion and drink within 1 day.

Deep Goodness Nettle Blend

 iron-rich | YIELDS 1 QUART

This nutrient-rich tonic infusion combines nettle with other nutritious herbs as well as herbs that are calming, balancing, and gentle on the nervous system. It's a deep nettle brew with highlights of flowers and memories of the garden. Sweeten this drink lightly with wildflower honey and enjoy it every day throughout the cold winter months.

2 tablespoons crumbled dried nettle leaves

2 tablespoons crumbled dried alfalfa

2 tablespoons shredded dried red clover blossoms

2 tablespoons crumbled dried lemon balm leaves

2 tablespoons crumbled dried holy basil (tulsi) leaves

Combine the herbs in a medium saucepan. Pour 1 quart of boiling water over the herbs and cover the pan. Allow to sit undisturbed for 4 to 8 hours, according to your taste. Strain, then return the infusion to the pan. Gently reheat and sweeten as desired. Store the hot tea in a Thermos, or refrigerate in a pitcher or glass jar for iced tea. Drink 2 to 4 cups throughout the day.

Garden Flower Infusion

 refreshing | YIELDS 1 QUART

Harvest your colorful garden flowers on the stem at their peak in the summer, and dry them on a screen or sheets of newsprint in a shady, well-ventilated area. Strip the leaves and flowers from the stems once they are crispy-dry, and store them together in a large glass jar. Your blend will then be ready whenever you want a bright, summer-flavored infusion.

1 to 2 cups mixed dried flowers and leaves, such as violet, chickweed, calendula, hyssop, rose, bee balm, and/or mint

Combine the flowers and leaves in a medium saucepan. Pour 1 quart of boiling water over the herbs and cover the pan. Allow to sit undisturbed for 4 to 8 hours, according to your taste. Strain, then return the infusion to the pan. Gently reheat and sweeten as desired. Store the hot tea in a Thermos, or refrigerate in a pitcher or glass jar for iced tea. Drink 2 to 4 cups throughout the day.

RED CLOVER
Trifolium pratense

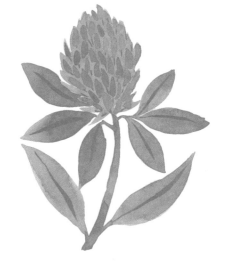

Valued both internally and externally to soothe eczema and psoriasis, red clover makes a useful compress for burns, weepy blisters, and rashes. Mid-nineteenth-century herbalist Samuel Thompson made it into a paste to treat skin cancers, and modern research suggests red clover may indeed exhibit antineoplastic, or tumor-inhibiting, activity. It contains phytoestrogens and phytosterols, compounds that make red clover valuable for menopausal women with hot flashes.

Historically, mineral-rich red clover has been considered a "blood cleanser," draining fluid from the lymphatic system, improving circulation, and helping the liver expel excess toxins. Acids build up in the lymph and blood, and Chinese herbalists refer to these toxins as "heat," which contributes to "hot" diseases. As an alterative, or an herb that assists the body in proper elimination of wastes, cooling red clover helps remove these toxins, dissolves external cysts, and aids in expectorant and antispasmodic formulas for bronchitis. Use naturally sweet red clover in teas, infusions, honeys, syrups, puddings, elixirs, vinegars, herb powder blends, and smoothies.

LICORICE
Glycyrrhiza glabra

Anise-flavored licorice root has long been popular as a remedy for respiratory congestion and digestive complaints. Taken for coughing, wheezing, catarrh build-up, and bronchitis for both children and adults, licorice is most delicious as a hot tea or syrup. Rich in glycosides (especially glycyrrhizin), saponins, flavonoids, bitter principles, volatile oil, coumarins, asparagine, and hormone-like estrogenic substances, licorice assists cases of peptic ulceration, gastritis, and ulcers, and it can treat colic or indigestion with great success. Its use for peptic and gastric ulcers is long-standing, as it has soothing demulcent effects and also directly promotes the production of healing prostaglandins. It also acts as a hepatic, stimulating the liver to manufacture bile. Use licorice root fresh or dried in teas, infusions, decoctions, syrups, herbal milks, herb powder blends, electuaries, and in small amounts in smoothies. Experiment with using a small amount in broths and soups if you like anise flavor.

Immune Tonic Decoction 1

 immune support | YIELDS 1 QUART

For an immune boost any time of year, sip on this pleasant-tasting and deeply healing decoction. These herbs are renowned for supporting the immune system (astragalus, licorice, and echinacea), stimulating blood flow throughout the body (ginger), fighting infection (echinacea, ginger, pau d'arco), and killing pathogens (pau d'arco). Add more licorice to the blend for a sweeter version of this mildly pleasant and straightforward beverage.

- 2 tablespoons dried chopped astragalus root
- 2 tablespoons dried chopped gingerroot
- 2 tablespoons dried chopped echinacea root
- 2 tablespoons dried chopped licorice root
- 1 tablespoon dried chopped pau d'arco bark

Combine the herbs and 1 quart of fresh cold water in a medium saucepan. Bring just to a boil over high heat. Reduce the heat to low, cover the pan, and simmer for 12 to 20 minutes, according to your taste. Strain into a Thermos and enjoy throughout the day.

Immune Tonic Decoction 2

 immune support | YIELDS 1 QUART

This immune-system-supporting decoction, tastes mintier, has a more pronounced garden flavor, and is not as medicinal tasting. All these herbs support the body during viral and bacterial infections. Adjust the licorice to taste. A shorter steeping time will bring out more of the thyme and mint flavors, and you'll get stronger flavors of elderberry and licorice if you steep it for longer.

- 2 tablespoons dried elderberries
- 2 tablespoons crumbled dried lemon balm leaves
- 2 tablespoons crumbled dried Saint-John's-wort leaves and flowers
- 2 tablespoons crumbled dried peppermint leaves
- 1 tablespoon dried thyme leaves
- 1 tablespoon dried licorice root, or to taste
- Honey, to taste

Combine the elderberries, lemon balm, Saint-John's-wort, peppermint, thyme, and licorice in a medium saucepan. Pour 1 quart fresh cold water over the herbs and bring just to a boil over high heat. Reduce the heat to low, cover the pan, and simmer for 12 to 20 minutes, according to your taste. Strain into a Thermos, sweeten with honey to taste, and enjoy throughout the day.

Dandelion Digestive Decoction

 digestive support | YIELDS 1 QUART

This strong, coffee-like drink is fortifying. It's a hearty drink that's fantastic for digestion, helpful for the bladder and urinary system because it is a diuretic, and soothing on a sore throat. It also presents quite a flavor profile: deep, satisfying, and rich, but given brightness and complexity by a hint of caraway. Start with the smaller quantity of caraway until you find the amount you like best.

2 to 4 tablespoons dried chopped dandelion root

2 to 4 tablespoons dried chopped chicory root

¼ to 1 teaspoon caraway seeds

Honey, to taste

Milk, to taste, optional

Combine the dandelion, chicory, and caraway in a medium saucepan. Pour 1 quart fresh cold water over the herbs and bring just to a boil over high heat. Reduce the heat to low, cover the pan, and simmer for 15 to 20 minutes, according to your taste. Strain into a Thermos, sweeten with honey to taste, and add milk if desired. Enjoy throughout the day.

DANDELION ROOT
Taraxacum officinale

Dandelion root is high in iron and can be eaten raw or cooked, or it can be dried and ground to be used like coffee, especially combined with dried chicory root. Its earthy flavor combines well with caraway, and it lends itself well to syrups. It is especially suited to vinegars, which efficiently extract its minerals; use strong vinegars such as apple cider or balsamic. Brew into a strong, dark beverage with chicory root and a tiny amount of sweetener.

6

CHAIS AND MULLING BLENDS

CHAIS AND MULLING BLENDS are traditionally complex and spicy blends of leaves, roots, barks, spices, and sometimes dried fruits that are steeped in water, milk, apple juice, lemonade, or even red wine. They have a great depth of flavor and can be very warming when served hot. The recipes here use herbs that are stimulant (such as ginger), heart supportive (such as hawthorn), and digestive (such as fennel).

Blend these herbs well in advance and store them in a glass jar with a tight lid; no refrigeration is necessary. Keep them nearby so you will be tempted to use them often; full of trace minerals, they have a rich flavor that makes sipping a drink on a cold night a special pleasure. The chai blends are heavenly steeped in a pot of dark-green nettle infusion, or steeped in water and then lightly sweetened and made creamy with the addition of whole milk. Enjoy the other blends steeped in hot apple cider, hot lemonade, or hot red wine. Steep the blends in the drink of your choice in a large open pot, strain into mugs or into a Thermos to keep hot, and serve with honey or milk as desired.

CHAI

Typically made with black tea, roots, seeds, and dried fruits, chai is often caffeinated and powerfully scented. Chais are meant to be steeped in water or milk, and many people add honey. The following recipes omit the caffeinated black tea and substitute other herbs with depth and complexity, such as rooibos, which results in caffeine-free chais that are soothing and satisfying.

Nettle Chai Blend

 energizing | YIELDS 1 QUART DRY CHAI BLEND

Pleasant and different, this blend combines green, nutritious nettles with the exotic spices we expect in a chai. It makes a cup that is fragrant, lightly sweet, and smooth on the tongue. You also get to enjoy the nutritional benefits of nettles without any of the caffeine typically found in chais.

3 cups crumbled dried nettle leaves

3 tablespoons dried chopped orange peel

2 tablespoons cinnamon chips, or one 3-inch stick, broken into pieces

1 tablespoon dried chopped gingerroot

2 teaspoons dried allspice berries

1 teaspoon cardamom seeds, or 12 whole pods

3 star anise pods, broken into pieces

Honey, to taste, optional

Milk, to taste, optional

Stir together the nettles, orange peel, cinnamon, ginger, allspice, cardamom, and anise in a medium bowl. Transfer to a 1-quart glass jar, cap, and label. Store on a pantry shelf until ready to use.

To brew a cup of chai, pour 1 cup of boiling water over 1 teaspoon of the herbal blend and let steep for 15 minutes. (Alternatively, brew in a percolator: for each cup of water, put 1 teaspoon herbal blend into the filter basket; brew for 15 to 20 minutes.) Strain into hot mugs and sweeten with honey and/or add milk to taste, if desired.

Deep Rooibos Chai Blend

 energizing | YIELDS 1 PINT DRY CHAI BLEND

Rooibos tea has become a favorite in recent years because it offers a rich and complex flavor and a boost in energy, yet it is caffeine-free. The flavor reminds me of hibiscus with more depth, or hawthorn with a little bitterness. It combines well with licorice and ginger, and in this blend it plays in the cup with deep ginger flavors and bright cardamom. I love to enjoy this heady, heavenly drink hot for a satisfying, fortifying feeling on a cold day. I find it doesn't need honey or milk, but these do add to its richness.

½ cup loose red rooibos tea

½ cup dried licorice root

½ cup dried chopped gingerroot

3 tablespoons dried chopped orange peel

2 teaspoons cinnamon chips

1 teaspoon cardamom seeds, or 12 whole pods

Honey, to taste, optional

Milk, to taste, optional

Stir together the rooibos, licorice, ginger, orange peel, cinnamon, and cardamom in a small bowl. Transfer to a 1-pint glass jar, cap, and label. Store on a pantry shelf until ready to use.

To brew a cup of chai, pour 1 cup of boiling water over 2 teaspoons of the herbal blend and let steep for 15 minutes. (Alternatively, brew in a percolator: for each cup of water, put 2 teaspoons of herbal blend into the filter basket; brew for 15 to 20 minutes.) Strain into a mug and sweeten with honey and/or add milk to taste, if desired.

Ashwagandha Chai by Kate Gilday

 calming | YIELDS ABOUT 1 PINT DRIED CHAI BLEND,
PLUS 1 CUP BREWED CHAI

Ashwagandha Chai is a warming beverage, excellent for those with slow or sluggish digestion. Herbalist Kate Gilday uses this delicious chai to nourish and calm others, and to help support restful sleep. "I have shared this formula with many clients who have found it invaluable as a sleep aid," says Kate. "It can be enjoyed on a daily or nightly basis, aiding both digestion and the nervous system." She also uses it to support the immune and endocrine systems.

Unlike the other chai recipes here, this recipe is made with warm milk (see more on the benefits of herbal milks, including how to make an herbal milk, on page 134). Drink a cup before bedtime to help with sleep, or drink a couple of cups throughout the day to help your endocrine, digestive, and immune systems.

FOR THE ASHWAGANDHA CHAI BLEND

8 ounces ashwagandha powder

2 tablespoons ground cardamom

1 tablespoon ground cinnamon

1 tablespoon ground ginger

FOR THE ASHWAGANDHA CHAI BEVERAGE

1 cup milk, such as fresh cow or goat milk (preferably raw) or coconut or other nut milk

1 teaspoon Ashwagandha Chai Blend

Pinch of freshly grated nutmeg

3 to 5 drops pure maple syrup, or 1 date, chopped, optional

To make the chai blend, stir together the ashwagandha, cardamom, cinnamon, and ginger in a small bowl. Transfer to a 1-pint glass jar, cap, and label. Store on a pantry shelf until ready to use.

To brew a cup of chai beverage, warm the milk in a small saucepan, covered, over low heat. Add 1 teaspoon of the chai blend and simmer gently over very low heat for 10 minutes. Pour into a cup or mug. Grate nutmeg over the drink and stir in maple syrup if desired.

MULLING BLENDS

Unlike chai blends, mulling spice blends are meant to be steeped in apple juice, lemonade, or red wine. They are best served hot, sometimes with a squeeze of lemon juice. Like chai, a mulling spice blend will stay fragrant and tasty for months when stored properly in an airtight glass jar on a pantry shelf.

Mulling Spice Blend

 digestive support | YIELDS ABOUT 1 QUART DRY MULLING BLEND, PLUS ABOUT ½ GALLON MULLED BEVERAGE

I love this traditional mulling spice blend steeped in a pot of apple cider. It combines all the exotic flavors of the spices with the comforting freshness of apples and results in a smooth, peppery mulled cider that is calming and soothing for the nervous system and for digestion. This blend can also be steeped in red wine.

FOR THE MULLING SPICE BLEND

- 1 cup cinnamon chips
- 1 cup dried chopped orange peel
- 1 cup dried chopped gingerroot
- ½ cup peppercorns
- ½ cup dried allspice berries
- ½ cup whole cloves
- 5 to 8 star anise pods
- ¼ cup cardamom pods
- ½ teaspoon clove oil, optional

FOR THE MULLED BEVERAGE

- ½ gallon apple cider, or 1.5 liters red wine
- 1 to 2 tablespoons Mulling Spice Blend
- Fresh orange slices or candied ginger, for garnish

To make the mulling blend, stir together the cinnamon, orange peel, ginger, peppercorns, allspice, cloves, star anise, and cardamom in a large bowl. Stir in the clove oil, if desired. Transfer to a 1-quart glass jar, cap, and label. Store on a pantry shelf until ready to use.

To brew a batch of mulled beverage, pour the apple cider or red wine into a large saucepan and add 1 to 2 tablespoons of the mulling blend. Bring to a boil over medium heat, then reduce the heat to low and simmer for 20 to 30 minutes. Strain and serve hot, garnished with fresh orange slices or candied ginger.

ROOIBOS
Aspalathus linearis

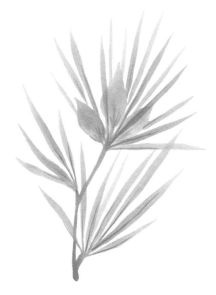

Native to South Africa, this shrub produces leaves that are fermented and dried and used in a way similar to black tea, but without the caffeine. When brewed, it tastes warm and rich and very comforting; it is antioxidant, mildly astringent, and has a lower tannin profile than black tea. Blend rooibos tea into chai blends for a delightful taste and warming, nourishing drink.

ASHWAGANDHA
Withania somnifera

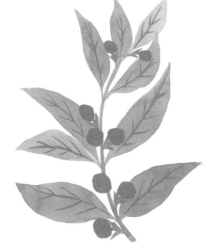

Ashwagandha is a small shrub native to India that produces small, reddish, astringent berries and has brown roots that are collected for medicine. Long a favorite herb in Ayurvedic medicine, ashwagandha is renowned as an anti-inflammatory and a tonic. It supports the immune system and is helpful when a person is recuperating from an illness. The root is tonic to the cardiovascular system and the female reproductive system. Because ashwagandha is also antispasmodic, Chinese/Cherokee/Western herbal practitioner David Winston suggests combining ashwagandha with black cohosh, kava, and wood betony to ease fibromyalgic pain. For a general male tonic, combine ashwagandha root with ginger, star anise, sarsaparilla root, gotu kola, and fenugreek. Because it helps reduce muscle spasm, it may be of help in Parkinson's disease. Because ashwagandha is relaxing (some say sedative), use it for nighttime teas, chai, and herbal milks.

Berry Good Hawthorn Mulling Blend

 heart support | YIELDS ABOUT 1 QUART DRY MULLING BLEND,
PLUS ½ GALLON MULLED BEVERAGE

This mulling blend for apple cider or lemonade brings out the best of wild berries. These berries are heart healthy and delicious and make a lovely, soothing beverage that can be sipped hot on cold nights.

FOR THE BERRY GOOD HAWTHORN MULLING BLEND

1 cup dried hawthorn berries

1 cup dried elderberries

1 cup dried rose hips

½ cup dried chopped lemon or orange peel

¼ cup dried allspice berries

¼ cup whole cloves

FOR THE MULLED BEVERAGE

½ gallon apple cider or lemonade

1 to 2 tablespoons Berry Good Hawthorn Mulling Blend

2 to 4 teaspoons sugar, optional

Fresh orange slices or candied ginger, for garnish

To make the mulling blend, stir together the hawthorn berries, elderberries, rose hips, lemon peel, allspice, and cloves in a large bowl. Transfer to a 1-quart glass jar, cap, and label. Store on a pantry shelf until ready to use.

To brew a batch of mulled beverage, pour the apple cider or lemonade into a large saucepan and add 1 to 2 tablespoons of the mulling blend and the sugar, if desired. Bring to a boil over medium heat, then reduce the heat to low and simmer for 20 to 30 minutes, stirring occasionally. Strain and serve hot, garnished with fresh orange slices or candied ginger.

Fennel Seed Steeping Blend

 digestive support | YIELDS ABOUT 1 QUART DRY MULLING BLEND,
PLUS ½ GALLON MULLED BEVERAGE

This unusual blend is actually a tasty and effective digestive aid. Steep in hot apple cider for a zippy and healthful treat on a cold night.

FOR THE FENNEL SEED STEEPING BLEND

1 cup fennel seeds

1 cup aniseeds

1 cup dried chopped gingerroot

½ cup dried chopped orange peel

¼ cup caraway seeds

FOR THE MULLED BEVERAGE

½ gallon apple cider or lemonade

1 to 2 tablespoons Fennel Seed Steeping Blend

2 to 4 tablespoons sugar, optional

Fresh orange slices or candied ginger, for garnish

To make the mulling blend, stir together the fennel seeds, anise seeds, ginger, orange peel, and caraway seeds in a large bowl. Transfer to a 1-quart glass jar, cap, and label. Store on a pantry shelf until ready to use.

To brew a batch of mulled beverage, pour the apple cider or lemonade into a large saucepan and add 1 to 2 tablespoons of the steeping blend and the sugar, if desired. Bring to a boil over medium heat, then reduce the heat to low and simmer for 20 to 30 minutes, stirring occasionally. Strain and serve hot, garnished with fresh orange slices or candied ginger.

ALLSPICE

Pimenta dioica

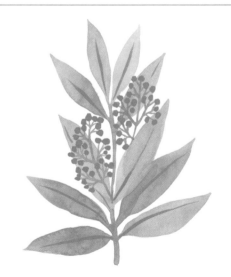

A spice in the true sense of the word, this little unripe berry often flavors confections and pastries, though my husband also adds it to his tomato sauce as his "secret ingredient." The berries are frequently paired with cinnamon and nutmeg, though they grow in different hemispheres. True allspice, which is native to the Caribbean and parts of Mexico, is different from the American allspice that herbalist Doug Elliott likes to use, which is harvested from the *Lindera benzoin* tree, which grows wild all over the eastern United States. Use allspice in small amounts to flavor foods and bring out a rich sweetness, or to counteract strongly peppery or acidic flavors.

Lemon Zinger Mulling Blend

 energizing | YIELDS ABOUT 1 QUART DRY MULLING BLEND,
PLUS ½ GALLON MULLED BEVERAGE

This is a zippy mulling blend, and it's great for getting the blood moving on a cold day. Come in from the snow and sit down to a hot mug of Lemon Zinger Mulled Apple Cider!

FOR THE LEMON ZINGER MULLING BLEND

1 cup dried chopped gingerroot

1 cup dried chopped lemon peel

½ cup dried chopped lemongrass

¼ cup dried hibiscus flowers

FOR THE MULLED BEVERAGE

½ gallon apple cider or lemonade

1 to 2 tablespoons Lemon Zinger Mulling Blend

2 to 4 tablespoons sugar, optional

Fresh lemon slices or candied ginger, for garnish

To make the mulling blend, stir together the ginger, lemon peel, lemongrass, and hibiscus in a large bowl. Transfer to a 1-quart glass jar, cap, and label. Store on a pantry shelf until ready to use.

To brew a batch of mulled beverage, pour the apple cider or lemonade into a large saucepan and add 1 to 2 tablespoons of the mulling blend and the sugar, if desired. Bring to a boil over medium heat, then reduce the heat to low and simmer for 15 to 20 minutes, stirring occasionally. Strain and serve hot, garnished with fresh lemon slices or candied ginger.

Berry Blue Mulling Blend

 nourishing | YIELDS ABOUT 1 QUART DRY MULLING BLEND,
PLUS ½ GALLON MULLED BEVERAGE

An antioxidant-rich combination of wild and cultivated berries and spices, this bright blend will enliven a pot of apple cider or revive a bottle of red wine. Complex and deep, it seems to fortify the blood from the inside out.

(Add the chaste-tree berries if you have them available and if you want to include this traditional women's herb for monthly balance.)

FOR THE BERRY BLUE MULLING BLEND

1 cup dried elderberries

1 cup dried cranberries

1 cup dried blueberries

½ cup dried allspice berries

½ cup peppercorns

1 cup dried goji berries, optional

1 cup chaste-tree berries, optional

FOR THE MULLED BEVERAGE

½ gallon apple cider or 0.5 liter red wine

1 to 2 tablespoons Berry Blue Mulling Blend

2 to 4 teaspoons sugar, optional

Fresh lemon slices or candied ginger, for garnish

To make the mulling blend, stir together the elderberries, cranberries, blueberries, allspice, peppercorns, and goji berries and chaste-tree berries (if using) in a large bowl. Transfer to a 1-quart glass jar, cap, and label. Store on a pantry shelf until ready to use.

To brew a batch of mulled beverage, pour the apple cider or red wine into a large saucepan and add 1 to 2 tablespoons of the mulling blend and the sugar, if desired. Bring to a boil over medium heat, then reduce the heat to low and simmer for 15 to 20 minutes, stirring occasionally. Strain and serve hot, garnished with fresh lemon slices or candied ginger.

Alternatively, brew this blend as a decoction by simmering 2 teaspoons of the herbal mixture per cup of boiling water for 12 to 15 minutes.

7

SMOOTHIES AND DELICIOUS DRINKS

IN ADDITION TO TEAS, CHAIS, and mulled beverages, so many drinks are perfect vehicles for delicious and nourishing medicinal herbs. Most herbs can be dried and powdered, making them excellent additions to fruit and vegetable smoothies. Powdered herbs also lend themselves easily to milkshakes and hot milk drinks, as well as to honey-based electuaries (see page 60). In this chapter, you'll also find a recipe for a tangy kombucha, as well as lemonades that burst with lemony flavor and vitamins and minerals. You'll also discover a fermented herbal soda that children find delicious and fresh juices in which fruits, vegetables, and herbs are all pressed together, creating vibrant tastes and colors. There's even a "coffee" made from foraged seeds.

Don't feel intimidated about using herbs in your favorite beverages—the quantities are very forgiving and can be adjusted easily. Experiment to find the flavors that suit you best, and use a variety of leaves, berries, and roots to experience all that medicinal herbs have to offer.

Smoothies of fresh or frozen fruit are refreshing on a hot day, or any time you need a burst of vitamins. All sorts of frozen fruit can be used to make a smoothie: bananas, guava, pomegranate, papaya, grapes, mango, pears, plums, cherries, apples, strawberries, raspberries, blueberries . . . the list goes on. Many people like to add spirulina or a store-bought protein powder to their smoothies, but it's just as easy and delicious to add a homemade herbal powder, which will provide antioxidants, vitamins, and the tonic goodness of traditional herbs. The smoothie blends you'll find here are meant to be combined as powders and added by the spoonful or scoop to your smoothies; also try adding them to hot milk or cold fruit juices.

To make your smoothie, use a powerful blender and include your favorite fruits. Add ice cubes if desired, and if it is too thick, add milk, yogurt, tea, juice, or water. Start with a small amount of powder and work your way up to achieve the flavor and effect you want.

How to Make an Herb Powder
To grind an individual herb into a powder, simply place a handful of dried herb in a coffee grinder and pulse. Strain the powder through a mesh sieve to remove unground pieces. (To purchase already-prepared single-herb powders, see Resources on page 232.) To create a blend, grind each herb individually, then stir the powders together. Store your powdered herb mix in a glass jar with a tight-fitting lid. Label it (Don't forget to label!), and keep your mix on the countertop within easy reach, so you will remember to include it in your daily smoothie, shake, or juice; mixes can also be added to oatmeal or sprinkled on yogurt and whisked into hot milk. As long as they stay dry, these powder blends will have a long shelf life.

There are as many powders as there are herbs. Almost any herb can be ground into a powder, and those that are nutritive, sustaining, and fortifying are the best to use in smoothies. Their flavors range from bland to dusky to tart. A sampling of herb powders on page 113 demonstrates what you can expect them to taste like in your smoothies:

THE FLAVORS AND BENEFITS OF BASIC HERB POWDERS

POWDERED HERB	FLAVOR PROFILE	BENEFITS
Amla or amalaki (*Phyllanthus emblica*)	Tart, mildly bitter	Nourishing
Ashwagandha (*Withania somnifera*)	Papery, bland, mildly bitter	Calming, stress support
Astragalus root (*Astragalus membranaceus*)	Pleasant, resin-like, a hint of tartness	Immune support
Calendula (*Calendula officinalis*)	Mildly bitter, pleasant	Immune support, digestive support
Elderberry (*Sambucus canadensis*)	Tart	Immune support
Fo-ti root (*Polygonum multiflorum*)	Bland	Immune support
Gingerroot (*Zingiber officinale*)	Sharp, peppery, hot	Immune support
Gotu kola (*Centella asiatica*)	Mildly bitter	Nourishing, stress support
Nettle (*Urtica dioica*)	"Green," bland	Nourishing, stress support, iron-rich
Oatstraw (*Avena sativa*)	Bland, pleasant	Nourishing, stress support, calming
Schizandra (*Schizandra chinensis*)	Bright, strongly tart, medicinal	Energizing
Shatavari root (*Asparagus racemosus*)	Pleasant, papery, resin-like	Energizing, promotes clarity & memory
Slippery elm (*Ulmus rubra*)	Dry, papery, mealy	Digestive support, calming, nourishing
Triphala blend: amla, or amalaki (*Phyllanthus emblica*, also known as *Emblica officianalis*); haritaki (*Terminalia chebula*); bibhitaki (*Terminalia belerica*)	Dry, tart, medicinal	Nourishing, stress support

CHASTE-TREE BERRY

Vitex agnus-castus

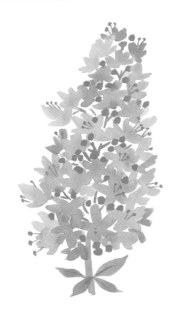

This pretty, small tree with deeply serrated leaves and purple flowers acquired its name from the Greeks, who, along with English monks and pagan priestesses, used the dried berries to suppress sexual desires during ceremonies and in cloister. Similarly, Arabic healers considered the berry and leaf to be calming.

Women today use the berries for entirely different purposes, often to *increase* libido. *Vitex* stimulates the pituitary gland, normalizing the progesterone and estrogen levels. Herbalists today recommend *Vitex* for women suffering from dysmenorrhea or premenstrual syndrome, and especially for menopausal women.

The dried berries, which resemble peppercorns, are rather tasteless, but they brew into a pleasant tea and can be added to chai blends.

Nerve-Building Milkshake

 stress support | YIELDS 2 TO 3 CUPS

Similar to a smoothie, this creamy milkshake "hides" the herbs so you don't even know they are there. These are tonic herbs, generally calming and supportive, and can be used long-term.

- 1 cup fresh cow or goat milk (preferably raw) or coconut or other nut milk
- 1 cup choppd packed fresh young nettle leaves
- 2 tablespoons chopped packed fresh young lemon balm leaves
- 1 teaspoon fo-ti powder
- 1 teaspoon gotu kola powder
- 1 teaspoon vervain powder

1 large frozen banana, peeled and frozen

½ cup raw almonds

1 tablespoon unsalted almond butter

½ teaspoon vanilla extract

2 cups water, plus more if needed

Honey, to taste, optional

At least an hour in advance, prepare the infused milk: Combine 1 cup of milk and the nettles and lemon balm in a small saucepan over medium heat. Bring to a light boil, then reduce the heat to low and simmer for 10 minutes. Remove the pan from the heat and allow the mixture to cool.

Strain the milk mixture into a blender. Add the fo-ti, gotu kola, and vervain powders and the banana, almonds, almond butter, vanilla extract, and water. Blend on high speed, adding more water as needed to reach your desired consistency. Blend honey to taste, if desired, and serve immediately.

Green Machine Smoothie

 nourishing | YIELDS ¼ CUP POWDER BLEND,
PLUS ABOUT 3 CUPS SMOOTHIE

A mineral-and-vitamin powerhouse, this smoothie mix is green, green, green. The green chlorophyll is mildly laxative, and nettles are mildly diuretic. Mixed with freshly frozen fruits in a smoothie, this blend is energizing and strengthening. It tastes earthy and deep, and it's good blended with frozen blueberries, mangoes, pears, plums, and bananas.

FOR THE GREEN MACHINE POWDER BLEND

1 tablespoon plus 1 teaspoon nettle powder

1 tablespoon plus 1 teaspoon alfalfa powder

1 tablespoon plus 1 teaspoon spirulina powder

FOR THE SMOOTHIE

2 cups frozen blueberries, mangoes, pears, plums, and/or bananas

1 to 2 cups apple juice or cider

1 rounded teaspoon Green Machine Powder Blend

To make the powder blend, stir together the herb powders in a small glass jar, then cap and label. Store on the countertop.

To make a smoothie, blend the frozen fruits and apple juice in a blender. Add 1 rounded teaspoon of the powder blend and blend well. Drink cold.

VERVAIN

Verbena hastata and *V. officinalis*

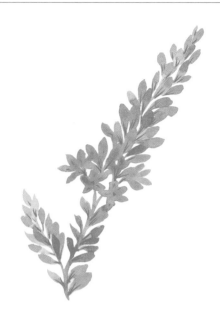

Not to be confused with lemon verbena, this small and easily overlooked flower has a long history in European legend and folklore; it said to have been included in love potions and cherished for bringing love and safety. Today, the herb is used medicinally, both as an herbal preparation and a homeopathic remedy, to treat nervous debility, exhaustion, overwork, and sleeplessness, although it is too mild to be a specific remedy for insomnia. Vervain eases premenstrual syndrome, fatigue at work as well as during childbirth, and stomach complaints due to anxiety. In teas its flavor is mild, nondescript, and pleasant.

ALFALFA

Medicago sativa

Although some people claim they feel like they are drinking horsefeed when they have alfalfa tea, it really has a mild, meadowy scent. Either way, they are doing their bodies good. Alfalfa is extremely high in minerals and a plethora of vitamins, and in addition to being healthy for people, for centuries it has been useful as forage for livestock. Cultures around the world have used cooling, fortifying alfalfa to address a range of health issues, and its benefits probably come primarily from its abundant nutrients. Blend alfalfa with other meadow herbs, including red clover, nettles, violets, and oats, for tea; it also blends well with the leaves and flowers of the linden tree, and with calendula flowers. Use powdered alfalfa in smoothie blends and electuaries.

Daily Tonic Smoothie

 clarity & memory | YIELDS ABOUT ¼ CUP POWDER BLEND,
PLUS ABOUT 3 CUPS SMOOTHIE

As an everyday tonic, this powder blend is a pleasant and enjoyable way to gain a little energy and nourish the mind and body. Mix it with mild or sweet fruits and add a little yogurt for a creamy, probiotic treat.

FOR THE DAILY TONIC POWDER BLEND

1 tablespoon plus 1 teaspoon amla powder

1 tablespoon plus 1 teaspoon gotu kola powder

2 teaspoons nettle powder

FOR THE SMOOTHIE

2 cups frozen bananas, plums, cherries, and/or peaches

1 to 2 cups apple juice

2 tablespoons yogurt, optional

1 rounded teaspoon Daily Tonic Powder Blend

To make the powder blend, stir together the herb powders in a small glass jar, then cap and label. Store on the countertop.

To make a smoothie, blend the frozen fruits and apple juice in a blender. Add the yogurt (if desired) and 1 rounded teaspoon of the powder blend and blend well. Drink cold.

Immunity Smoothie

 immune support | YIELDS ABOUT ¼ CUP POWDER BLEND,
PLUS ABOUT 3 CUPS SMOOTHIE

This blend of immune-supporting herbs has a strong and pronounced, but not unpleasant, medicinal flavor and is good mixed with strong-tasting fruits such as pineapple, grapefruit, and orange.

FOR THE IMMUNITY POWDER BLEND

1 tablespoon plus 1 teaspoon echinacea root powder

1 tablespoon plus 1 teaspoon astragalus powder

2 teaspoons elderberry powder

1 teaspoon licorice root powder

FOR THE SMOOTHIE

> 2 cups frozen pineapple, grapefruit, and/or oranges
>
> 2 cups pineapple juice
>
> 1 rounded teaspoon Immunity Powder Blend

To make the powder blend, stir together the herb powders in a small glass jar, then cap and label. Store on the countertop.

To make a smoothie, blend the frozen fruits and pineapple juice in a blender. Add 1 rounded teaspoon of the powder blend and blend well. Drink cold.

Digestive Smoothie

 digestive support | YIELDS ⅛ CUP POWDER BLEND, PLUS ABOUT 2 CUPS SMOOTHIE

This blend has a strong, naturally sweet-tart flavor and is good mixed with fruits such as pineapple, apple, and strawberries. Alternatively, stir 1 teaspoon of this blend into 1 cup of hot milk and enjoy it as a hot drink. It is also good stirred into ¼ cup honey and spread on toast or eaten straight from the spoon.

FOR THE DIGESTIVE POWDER BLEND

> 2 teaspoons ground fennel seeds
>
> 2 teaspoons ground fenugreek seeds
>
> ½ teaspoon triphala powder

FOR THE SMOOTHIE

> 1 cup frozen pineapple, apple, and/or strawberries
>
> 1 cup apple juice or other fruit juice
>
> 1 rounded teaspoon Digestive Powder Blend

To make the powder blend, stir together the ground fennel seeds, ground fenugreek seeds, and triphala powder in a small glass jar. Cap and label, and store on the countertop.

To make a smoothie, blend the frozen fruits and apple juice in a blender. Add 1 rounded teaspoon of the powder blend and blend well. Drink cold.

Wild Berry Energy Smoothie

 energizing | YIELDS ABOUT ¼ CUP POWDER BLEND,
PLUS ABOUT 2 CUPS SMOOTHIE

This is a strongly flavored, fruity mix of powdered herbs that tastes tart and tangy and looks vibrantly pink. Blend this with apple cider and/or pineapple juice to let the tartness shine through. Full of antioxidants and vitamins, this smoothie makes for an uplifting and healthy start to your day.

FOR THE WILD BERRY ENERGY POWDER BLEND

2 teaspoons schizandra berry powder

2 teaspoons goji berry powder

2 teaspoons elderberry powder

2 teaspoons hawthorn berry powder

1 teaspoon hibiscus powder

1 teaspoon ground lemon peel

FOR THE SMOOTHIE

1 small fresh or frozen banana

½ cup frozen mango chunks

1 cup black currant or pineapple juice

1 rounded teaspoon Wild Berry Energy Powder Blend

To make the powder blend, stir together the herb powders and ground lemon peel in a small glass jar. Cap and label, and store on the countertop.

To make a smoothie, put the banana, mango, and black currant juice into a blender and blend to the desired consistency. Add 1 rounded teaspoon of the powder blend and blend well. Drink cold.

Brain Tonic Smoothie

 clarity & memory | YIELDS ABOUT ¼ CUP POWDER BLEND,
PLUS ABOUT 3 CUPS SMOOTHIE

Peppy and strong-flavored, this blend of culinary herbs can be used to keep you alert: the herbs are traditionally used to support cognitive function and memory. A small dose of this powder blend probably won't cause much of an effect, but using it daily over the long-term will improve

ELDER

Sambucus spp., especially *Sambucus nigra* and *Sambucus canadensis*

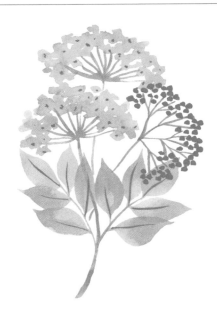

A magical and mystical plant, this small tree has been included (for better or worse) in European mythology and folktales for centuries. Because it has edible, medicinal, and functional uses, the elder tree has pressed itself into the lives of humans at every turn, earning it both the respect and fear of cultures and communities who have passed down their favorite, sometimes quirky, ways to use its berries, flowers, branches, and leaves. For our purposes, we can focus on its edible flowers— which are traditionally infused or extracted to help lower fevers, especially in infants and children, and to reduce upper respiratory congestion—and its edible berries, which are delicious cooked and, when processed, become immune-modulating, fever-reducing, anti-catarrhal, and astringent.

Elder's pale, creamy-colored umbels are a favorite of mothers, who use elder flower preparations to dry mucous secretions, soothe tender noses, and reduce fever. Considered safe and effective for babies and children, it is a key fever remedy. Make fritters with the fresh flower heads, or sprinkle them on salads. Use them fresh or dried in teas, infusions, honeys, and especially syrups—and don't worry if some stay behind in your honeys and syrups: they're beautiful suspended in the jar and are perfectly edible.

Elderberries are prized for reducing fever and supporting the immune system against viral, bacterial, and fungal infections. Berries will not form on the branch from which you harvested flowers, so it's best to specify some elder trees for flower harvest and other trees for berry harvest. Press the fresh berries into a glass jar and cover with apple cider vinegar. Use the dried berries in teas, infusions, honeys, and syrups, or powder the dried berries for use in smoothie blends. Fresh and dried berries can be used for soups and broths. (Caution: Elder leaves, stalks, and roots are not edible; only the flowers and berries are edible.)

blood flow, especially to the brain. Because of its strong flavor, mix it with strong-flavored juices such as pineapple and grapefruit. Alternatively, stir a spoonful into Citrus Yogurt (page 155) or try it in a chilled glass of tomato juice.

FOR THE BRAIN TONIC POWDER BLEND

> 1 tablespoon plus 1 teaspoon lemon balm powder
>
> 1 tablespoon plus 1 teaspoon peppermint powder
>
> ¼ teaspoon sage powder
>
> 2 teaspoons ground fennel seeds

FOR THE SMOOTHIE

> 2 cups frozen berries, such as blueberries or strawberries
>
> ½ frozen banana
>
> 1 cup juice, such as pomegranate, blueberry, or acai berry
>
> 1 rounded teaspoon Brain Tonic Powder Blend

To make the powder blend, stir together the herb powders and ground fennel seeds in a small glass jar. Cap and label, and store on the countertop.

To make a smoothie, put the berries, banana, and juice into a blender and blend. Add 1 rounded teaspoon of the powder blend and blend well. Drink cold.

Mind of the Goddess Smoothie

 clarity & memory | YIELDS ABOUT ⅓ CUP POWDER BLEND,
PLUS ABOUT 2 CUPS SMOOTHIE

Another brain tonic powder, this is a milder-tasting blend using Ayurvedic herbs, and it's delicious. It's become my favorite powder blend, and I use it frequently mixed into a cup of hot apple cider or milk as well as tossed into the blender whenever I'm making a fruit smoothie. I also stir it into my morning oatmeal. It's so mild it doesn't seem to impart any flavor, and its effects are actually quite noticeable. I feel steady and calm after drinking this, and I enjoy giving myself a little boost of goodness along with my breakfast.

SCHISANDRA
Schisandra chinensis

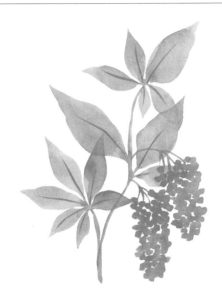

Appreciated in much the same way as
the leaves of true tea, the berries of
this plant give energy and help relieve
fatigue and exhaustion, but it contains
no caffeine. It is a flavorful berry; in fact,
it is known as "five-taste fruit" for the
fact that some people can discern all
five tastes of Chinese herbalism: sour,
sweet, bitter, acrid, and salty. It has been
a favorite remedy in China and Russia,
where it is enjoyed as a tea, a fruit juice,
a powder, and a syrup. Herbalist David
Winston calls it a "powerful adaptogen,
strengthening hypothalamic/pituitary/
adrenal function and normalizing nervous system and immune activity."
Use it when you feel fatigued or you have an athletic goal to reach, and
meditate on the quality of tasting many of life's flavors at once.

TRIPHALA

This is not one herb but rather a combination of the fruits of three trees: amalaki,
or amla (*Emblica officinalis*), bibhitaki (*Terminalia bellirica*), and haritaki (*Terminalia chebula*). Together, these fruits form a central part of the Ayurvedic formulary,
where this blend is used primarily to support the immune system and the digestive system. The blend is antioxidant and anti-inflammatory, making it popular for
inflammatory digestive upset. The flavor of the powder is dry, tart, and strong—
somewhat astringent but not unpleasant. Use this powder in honeys, hot herbal
milks, and smoothie blends.

CHINESE BOXTHORN (GOJI BERRY)
Lycium chinense

Delicious and tangy, this Chinese fruit has become popular in the West in dried
form for its lovely flavor and bright, beautiful red color. It's also popular because,
like many other dried fruits, goji berries can be eaten raw, out of hand. High in vitamins and minerals, goji berries make a good addition to granolas and cereals; they
can be powdered and used in smoothies; and they can be brewed in tea blends.
Their taste is similar to hibiscus flowers, and they are generally used as a flavoring
and added nutrient. Avoid if pregnant or nursing and when suffering from a cold
or the flu.

FOR THE MIND OF THE GODDESS POWDER BLEND

1 tablespoon plus 1 teaspoon shatavari powder

1 tablespoon plus 1 teaspoon ashwagandha powder

1 tablespoon plus 1 teaspoon amla powder

1 teaspoon fo-ti powder

1 teaspoon holy basil (tulsi) powder

½ teaspoon ginkgo powder

FOR THE SMOOTHIE

1 cup frozen peaches, pears, cherries, and/or mango

1 cup apple juice

1 rounded teaspoon Mind of the Goddess Powder Blend

To make the powder blend, stir together the herb powders in a small glass jar, then cap and label. Store on the countertop.

To make a smoothie, blend together the frozen fruits and apple juice in a blender. Add 1 rounded teaspoon of the powder blend and blend well. Drink cold.

Body of the Goddess Smoothie

 nourishing | YIELDS LESS THAN ¼ CUP POWDER BLEND,
PLUS ABOUT 3 CUPS SMOOTHIE

Like the Mind of the Goddess powder blend, this blend uses mild-tasting herbs to create a pleasant and nourishing treat. The nettle makes it slightly green. Shatavari is renowned in India as a "women's" herb, useful for digestive and reproductive issues. Treat yourself to a smoothie or juice enhanced with this blend after a workout or a hike in the woods. This is also nice mixed into a cup of hot milk after a day of snow play or skiing.

FOR THE BODY OF THE GODDESS POWDER BLEND

1 tablespoon plus 1 teaspoon amla fruit powder

1 tablespoon plus 1 teaspoon nettle powder

1 teaspoon shatavari powder

FOR THE SMOOTHIE

1 cup frozen mango, banana, blackberries, or blueberries

2 cups apple juice

1 rounded teaspoon Body of the Goddess Powder Blend

To make the powder blend, stir together the herb powders in a small glass jar, then cap and label. Store on the countertop.

To make a smoothie, blend together the frozen fruits and apple juice in a blender. Add 1 rounded teaspoon of the powder blend and blend well. Drink cold.

MORE DELICIOUS DRINKS

Sometimes our healing drinks need a little pizzazz. For example, fermenting herbs can give a beverage the extra enzymes it needs to help stimulate digestion, and they make kombuchas and herbal sodas delicious. Percolating an herb along with your coffee—such as persimmon seeds or chicory root—gives it a nutritious and flavorful boost, and it is so easy to do: just brew it all in an old-fashioned percolator over a woodstove or on the stove top—it's a great reason to visit the antique store! (Modern coffeemakers work well, too.)

The special drinks in this section can be enjoyed as treats or as daily beverages. Some support the digestive system, others the cardiovascular system. All are delicious, making it worth the extra effort to learn a new recipe. Some of them may become your favorites!

GINKGO

Ginkgo biloba

One of the most ancient trees, the ginkgo has been used in traditional medicine throughout China for more than a thousand years. Popularly used to enhance the memory, its effects are believed to stem from its ability to inhibit the reuptake of norepinephrine and from its cerebro-stimulatory traits. Ginkgo extracts have been shown in trials to elevate the mood, helpful for depression. It contains the flavonoid quercetin, a potent free radical scavenger, which, according to the National Institutes of Health, has been shown to reduce the severity of senile macular degeneration. Use ginkgo as a preventive tonic for supporting cognitive function, both short-term and long-term, in teas, infusions, herb powder blends, and smoothie blends.

Ginger Kombucha by Jan Buhrman

Kombucha is a fermented beverage usually made with black or green tea. The fermentation process involves introducing a culture of beneficial bacteria and yeast to a container of freshly brewed, cooled tea and feeding the culture sugar so that the entire container becomes fermented. The beverage is then refrigerated, where it continues to ferment, naturally building up carbonation and an intense flavor.

You'll notice this recipe calls for a scoby, a "symbiotic *colony of bacteria* and *yeast*." Kombucha is brewed under carefully controlled conditions so that the microorganisms that develop are helpful gut organisms that improve digestion and keep us healthy. A scoby, which is usually cream-colored and has the size and shape of a rubbery pancake, can be obtained from a friend who makes kombucha or from a mail-order source (see Resources on page 232). Be sure to use a large jar or container with roughly the same diameter as the scoby. Scobys can be used multiple times, and they produce "offspring," miniature scobys that can be used to start a new batch.

"I have tried this ginger kombucha several ways," says Kitchen Porch caterer and chef Jan Buhrman. "I like to add the ginger after making the kombucha because otherwise the scoby will take on the flavor of the ginger, which is fine if you will be making only ginger kombucha in the future." When choosing the sugar, select cane juice crystals or plain white sugar. Avoid brown or raw cane sugar, as these produce a "yeasty" result, and do not use maple syrup, honey, or artificial sweeteners, as these will create inconsistent and unreliable results.

1 gallon water

¼ cup black tea leaves

¼ cup plus 2 tablespoons green tea leaves

2 cups white sugar

3 cups premade unflavored kombucha beverage
(from your last homemade batch or store-bought)

Large glass jar the same diameter as your scoby (1½ gallon capacity),
for initial fermentation

1 scoby about 1 inch thick

3-inch piece of fresh gingerroot

Six 1-pint canning jars with lids or swing-top bottles

Bring the water to a boil in a medium stainless steel pot. As soon as the water boils, remove the pot from the heat and add the black tea, green tea, and sugar and stir well. Allow to steep until the tea has cooled to room temperature. Strain the tea into the large fermenting jar. Stir in the premade kombucha. Wash your hands, and then gently pick up the scoby and place it in the jar, where it will likely float on top of the tea. Cover the opening of the jar with a few layers of cheesecloth or a thin dish towel and secure with a rubber band.

Place the jar of fermenting kombucha out of direct sunlight and allow it to ferment at room temperature for 7 to 10 days, checking the kombucha and the scoby periodically. The culture should float to the top and the liquid will begin to ferment. Taste it after 5 days to see if it is tangy and bubbly. The amount of time needed will depend on how big the culture is and the temperature of the room. The warmer the room (especially at temperatures above 70°F), the faster the beverage will ferment, and it will continue to get tangier as the days go by. Jan notes, however, that eventually the ferment will reach its limit, and additional fermentation will result only in vinegar. The ideal time to stop the fermentation process is generally between 7 and 10 days.

On day 7, check the kombucha again for taste; when it tastes good to you, the kombucha is ready.

Carefully lift the scoby out of the jar, and either use it immediately to begin the process again, in another jar, or allow it to "rest" until you are ready to begin again. To let your scoby rest, keep it refrigerated in a jar with tea and sugar. Since every scoby is different in size, Jan suggests the following guideline: if your scoby is 4 inches in diameter and 2 inches thick, place it in a jar with 4 cups of cooled tea blended with 1 cup of sugar, and wrap the top of the jar with a cheesecloth. Check periodically to make sure the scoby is covered by the liquid, and store it for up to 4 months at an ideal temperature between 39°F and 50°F.

Brew 3 cups of tea, stir in 1 cup of sugar, and let cool, then add the scoby. Set aside and refrigerate 3 cups of the fermented kombucha to use as the premade starter tea in your next batch.

Scrub the ginger clean, but do not peel it. Grate it finely on a microplane or blend in a blender with a little kombucha. Divide the ginger evenly among the 6 glass jars. Fill the jars with fermented kombucha, leaving an inch of headspace, and cap.

Store the bottled kombucha at room temperature, out of direct sunlight, until carbonated, 1 to 3 days. Once carbonated, chill the kombucha in the refrigerator for at least 4 hours. Store in the refrigerator for up to several weeks.

GINGER
Zingiber officinale

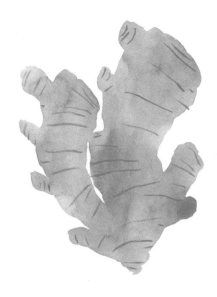

This favorite among spices, *Zingiber officinale* is a circulatory stimulant and is diaphoretic—that is, induces sweating to reduce high fevers. Called "pepper root," ginger stimulates digestive function, and people throughout history have brewed it with elderberry or mint to relieve morning sickness and motion sickness. It is used for cramps and nausea associated with premenstrual syndrome or pregnancy, and a poultice of shredded ginger or a compress of ginger tea eases arthritic pain and spasm. Herbalists use ginger internally to treat colds, bronchial ailments, and stomach complaints, and it is used on children's chests for colds.

Peel and chop ginger coarsely to add to stir-fries and Thai dishes. Make a weak ginger tea and use it in place of the water when cooking rice for an Oriental meal. Toss a slice of ginger in with beans while they're soaking or precooking, as it will make them more digestible. Candy peeled ginger slices by lightly steaming them and then dipping them in a simple sugar syrup. Use ginger liberally when you make herbal syrups, teas, decoctions, broths, soups, skillet dishes, and vinegars, keeping in mind that it is generally warming and stimulating. Use it powdered in hot herbal milks and electuaries. Use caution if gallstones are present and during pregnancy, and keep ginger use to a minimum during and after the first trimester.

Sumac "Lemonade"

YIELDS ABOUT 1 GALLON

Harvesting deep red sumac berries is a delicious endeavor. I love licking my fingers after plucking the fruit head off the stalk—the berries are covered with tangy acids (such as ascorbic and malic acids) that taste like lemon juice, and they make a tangy, tart, refreshing end-of-summer drink. Brew this into a hot tea and then refrigerate to make a strong lemonade, or plunge the berries into a pot of cold or room-temperature water and let them soak. Add lemon juice, if desired, but go light to allow the flavor of the sumac to shine through.

1 gallon water

6 to 8 fresh large heads of sumac berries (or 4 to 5 cups dried sumac berries)

Honey, maple syrup, sugar (for hot method), or sugar syrup (for cold method), optional

To brew in hot water: In a medium pot, bring the water to a boil. Add the sumac berries (or entire fruit heads), turn off the heat, and cover. Let sit for 3 minutes, then taste. If it is not yet strong enough, let it sit 1 or 2 minutes longer. As soon as it has a strong lemony flavor, strain into a pitcher. Don't let it brew too long—it will get bitter if brewed more than a few minutes. Compost the berries. Sweeten, if desired. Let cool to room temperature, then transfer to the refrigerator. Serve cold.

To brew in cold water: Fill a medium pot with cool or room-temperature water. Plunge the berries (or the entire fruit heads) into the pot. Rub the berries with your hands, or use a wooden spoon to agitate the water; this is to release the flavorful acids from the surface of the berries. Allow the berries to soak until the flavor is the strength you desire, about 10 minutes. Strain into a pitcher and add sweetener, if desired. Store in the refrigerator and serve cold.

Rose Petal Pink Lemonade
by Jan Berry

 refreshing | YIELDS 1 PINT INFUSED VINEGAR, PLUS 2 CUPS LEMONADE

Hobby farmer and *Nerdy Farm Wife* blogger Jan Berry makes this rosy lemonade at her home in the Blue Ridge Mountains of Virginia. She adds rose petal vinegar to a batch of fresh homemade lemonade, creating a deliciously tart and colorful drink she says children and adults adore. Plan ahead for the vinegar: you'll need to harvest the rose petals and begin infusing it about 2 weeks before you make this lemonade.

FOR THE ROSE PETAL VINEGAR

2 to 3 cups packed fresh rose petals

2 cups apple cider vinegar or white wine vinegar

FOR THE LEMONADE

½ cup freshly squeezed lemon juice

½ cup cane sugar, or ¼ cup honey

1½ cups water

1 to 5 teaspoons Rose Petal Vinegar

To make the vinegar, fill a 1-pint glass jar with the rose petals and pour in the vinegar. Gently swirl the jar to release air bubbles, cap tightly with a nonmetallic lid, and tuck away in a dark cupboard for about 2 weeks. Depending on the color of your roses, the vinegar will turn a lovely shade of pink or deep red. Strain. Store the infused vinegar in a clean, labeled jar or bottle in a cool, dark place for up to 1 year. (Keeping it out of direct sunlight will preserve the color.)

To make the lemonade, put the lemon juice and sugar into a large glass or quart jar and stir well to combine. Add the water and stir. Add the vinegar, 1 teaspoon at a time, until you reach the desired color and flavor. Add more sweetener, if needed. Chill in the refrigerator and serve cold.

Oxygenator Juice with Dill

by Sharon Egan and Manya Williams

 nourishing | YIELDS ABOUT 1½ CUPS

Juicing entrepreneurs Sharon Egan and Manya Williams launched their JuiceWell brand on both U.S. coasts, blending fresh-pressed fruit juices with herbs to create the healthiest drinks possible. Here they share two of their creations, which you can replicate using any small kitchen juicer. Use the freshest produce possible, unpeeled, and fresh herbs.

2 medium carrots

1 medium cucumber

1 medium beet

Small bunch of fresh dill

Wash all the produce. Juice each ingredient separately, including the dill with the beet, then combine the juices in a glass. Chill before drinking.

Renew Juice with Mint
by Sharon Egan and Manya Williams

 refreshing | YIELDS ABOUT 1½ CUPS

A refreshing juice-and-herb blend made with a juicer, this drink is packed with vitamin C from the raw Swiss chard, apple, and lemon. Chard also provides iron, calcium, and vitamin A, making this a nutritious wake-up beverage to serve chilled with a sprig of mint.

1½ apples

1 bunch of chard

1 lemon

Small bunch of fresh spearmint or peppermint

Wash all the produce. Juice each ingredient separately, including the mint with the lemon, then combine the juices in a glass. Chill before drinking.

Strong Roots: A Lacto-Fermented Herbal Soda
by Suzanna Stone

 digestive support | YIELDS ½ GALLON

Well known at herbalist gatherings for her delicious recipes—including homemade wines and sodas—Suzanna Stone works to bring the power of herbal medicine back to the people. She directs Owlcraft Healing Ways in central Virginia and teaches traditional foodways and healing arts. Here, she shares how to use wild, flavorful roots to create a fantastic lacto-fermented beverage that can be enjoyed by all ages as a soda.

Creating natural sodas is a wonderful way to get the extra enzymes and bacteria your body needs. Lactic acid bacteria (LAB) such as *Lactobacillus* convert the sugars in food to lactic acid, creating an acidic environment in the food that inhibits spoilage. According to the National Institutes of Health, LAB confers many benefits to the human body, including controlling intestinal infections, improving nutrition, facilitating digestion of lactose, and maintaining serum cholesterol levels. What's more, these fermented sodas taste delicious.

To obtain whey, Suzanna suggests putting 1 quart of stirred, whole milk yogurt into a colander or large fine-mesh strainer that has been lined with several layers of cheesecloth. Place the colander over a deep bowl, cover, and refrigerate for 15 to 24 hours. The liquid that drips from the yogurt is whey, which is high in enzymes and beneficial bacteria. Remove the colander and bowl from the refrigerator, then gather the edges of the cheesecloth into a bundle and secure them together with a rubber band. Slide a long-handled wooden spoon under the rubber band and suspend the bundle over the bowl for another 3 to 4 hours. When all the liquid whey has dripped from the bundle, scrape the solids from the cheesecloth; this is yogurt "cheese," which is like a tangy cream cheese. Add fresh or dried chopped herbs to this cheese and use it as a savory spread, or add it to smoothies. Suzanna also suggests enjoying it as a thick, Greek-style yogurt topped with fresh fruit. Pour the liquid whey into a jar. One quart of yogurt will yield about 2 cups of whey. Store tightly covered in the refrigerator for up to 6 months.

1 tablespoon dried chopped dandelion root

1 tablespoon dried chopped burdock root

1 tablespoon dried chopped sarsaparilla

1 tablespoon dried chopped licorice root

1 tablespoon grated fresh gingerroot

2 quarts water

1 cup yogurt whey

½ cup local honey

Juice of ½ lemon

Put the dandelion, burdock, sarsaparilla, licorice, ginger, and water into a large saucepan over high heat. Bring to a boil, then reduce the heat to low and simmer until the plant material falls to the bottom of the pan, 10 to 15 minutes. Strain into a large bowl and let cool to room temperature.

Stir together the whey, honey, and lemon juice in a ½-gallon jar. Fill the jar to the top with the cooled root tea (hot tea would kill the cultures in the whey). Stir until the honey is completely dissolved. Cover the jar tightly, and place on a plate on the countertop to ferment for 1 to 4 days. When the first very small amount of liquid seeps out of the jar, it is ready for the next step. The fermentation time will depend on the temperature of your kitchen: quicker in a warm kitchen, slower in a cool kitchen.

When the initial fermentation stage is complete, the mixture is ready to bottle. This secondary stage of fermentation builds carbonation, because carbon dioxide is one of the by-products of fermentation. Strain the fermented mixture into bottles, making sure to leave 2 inches of headspace to allow room for carbonation to build, and cap very tightly. Good bottles to use are screw-top sparkling water bottles, bail-cap bottles, or, if you have a bottle capper, small glass soda bottles.

Place the filled and capped bottles on the countertop to ferment further for another 2 to 4 days, until you notice that a very slight amount of the soda has seeped out. This indicates that carbonation has occurred. Generally, Suzanna says, as long as the temperature has stayed relatively constant, you can use the length of the initial fermentation as a guideline to determine how long the second stage of fermentation will last. In other words, if the initial fermentation took 2 days, it is reasonable to assume that this second stage of fermentation in the bottles will also take 2 days. Transfer to the refrigerator and store for up to 3 months. Drink cold anytime.

Persimmon Seed Coffee by Doug Elliott

Wild naturalist Doug Elliott suggests a variety of ways to use the pulp of persimmons: as a spread for bread, as an ice cream topping, substituted for bananas in your favorite banana-nut bread recipe, and even swirled in a parfait glass with whipped cream to make an elegant dessert. But don't throw out those seeds! Make Doug's fresh and fragrant (and caffeine-free) Persimmon Seed Coffee to enjoy alongside the delicious fruity desserts.

Preheat the oven to 325°F. Collect the seeds from your recent harvesting foray under the persimmon trees. Wash the remaining pulp off the seeds and roast them on a baking sheet until they are very dark brown. Crack a seed to be sure it's roasted all the way through. Allow the seeds to cool completely. At this point, you can transfer them whole to an airtight glass jar, or grind them and store the grounds in a jar. Cap, label, and store the jar in the pantry.

When you're ready to make "coffee," grind the seeds in a blender or coffee grinder if they are still whole and prepare as you would normal coffee: use 1 to 2 tablespoons of grounds per 6 ounces of water.

8

HOT HERBAL MILKS

"The land of milk and honey" refers to a mystical and enchanting place where dreams come true and all things are lovely. It's a wonderful image—both in literature and in the kitchen. If you can drink dairy milk without a problem and you enjoy its creamy texture and the many wonderful foods that can be made from it, or if you enjoy rice, almond, or soy "milk," you should certainly try using it with herbs to create remedies for fantastic nutrition.

Largely ignored in Western herbal medicine, combining milk and herbs is a wonderful back-to-the-land way to craft herbal remedies: you need not depend on external suppliers for the materials commonly used to make liquid herbal compounds that will be taken orally, such as vegetable glycerin and grain alcohol. Like water, milk can draw compounds from herbal matter to be readily absorbed by the body for increased nutrition. (Grain alcohol does extract many more medicinal compounds than milk will; the use of milk with herbs—especially in Ayurvedic formulas—is less about extracting compounds from plants and more about balancing the person's constitution.) In the following recipes, we are using the milk primarily as a nutritive vehicle; we will be adding powdered herbs to the milk to create the desired remedies.

Here's where we see the beauty of milk as a vehicle for herbs. In Ayurveda, hot milk is an integral component in the daily diet, appearing in both vegetarian and meat-based diets alongside beans, vegetables, fruit, and liquid drinks, and in the ancient Ayurvedic philosophy of life and health, milk is consumed warm or hot and infused with herbs and spices to make wonderfully nourishing remedies. Warm or hot milk is considered helpful for balancing vata and pitta tendencies, which generally exhibit as hot and dry; however, people who exhibit kapha (cold and heavy) tendencies should generally avoid dairy products. "Cow's milk is cold, heavy, sweet, and slimy, so it promotes kapha excess if taken cold," say authors Karta Purkh Singh Khalsa and Michael Tierra in *The Way of Ayurvedic Herbs*. However, "when cow's milk is heated and taken warm, it breaks down the long-chain proteins that are difficult to pass through the liver. Thus it seems to not cause the adverse congesting effects of cold, unprocessed liquid milk." In fact, in the Ayurvedic tradition milk is virtually *never* taken cold except as yogurt, where it is presumably somewhat predigested. Tonic herbs such as powdered ashwagandha, shatavari, ginger, and ginseng are traditionally taken in just-scalded warm milk and sweetened with a bit of honey; however, for many of the following recipes adding sweetener is unnecessary.

The following recipes are meant to encourage you to get more herbs into your diet. Although raw, unpasteurized fresh cow milk is best, these can be made with any milk, including nut milks. If you love to eat a bowl of fresh, creamy yogurt with your breakfast, try using the following powder blends to make your already-healthy yogurt even more flavorful and beneficial (see How to Make an Herbal Yogurt on page 151).

How to Make a Hot Herbal Milk

Pour ½ cup of milk into a small saucepan over medium heat. If using fresh herbs, such as grated fresh ginger or chopped fresh nettles, add them as soon as the milk is warm (if using herb powders, wait to add them). Continue to heat the milk or milk-and-herb mixture, stirring constantly, until it reaches the scalding point—the point just before boiling, when tiny bubbles first appear along the edges. Immediately remove the pan from the heat. (Heating the milk beyond this point can destroy vital enzymes, but heating just to the scalding point breaks down the long-chain proteins while keeping most of these enzymes intact.) If using herb powder, whisk ¼ to 1 teaspoon into the milk (¼ teaspoon for a mild remedy, 1 teaspoon

BURDOCK

Arctium lappa

This enormous wildflower (I've seen it reach 13 feet tall) has an equally enormous root that can have a diameter spanning six inches. It's incredibly difficult to dig out of the ground once it's established, but its persistent quality hints at its efficacy. Burdock produces a number of parts useful as both food and medicine. The seeds (these are the ones that stick to your socks and were the inspiration for Velcro) and the root are tinctured and used internally to treat acne. This plant is a supreme alterative, assisting the liver in its functions of metabolizing waste and regenerating red blood cells; it is frequently used as a "spring tonic" for "cleansing" the blood and liver. Burdock is used for lymph issues, "stagnant" illnesses, and especially to help clear skin infection and breakouts from the inside. The root can be sliced and boiled or sautéed and is a traditional food throughout Asia, known as *gobo*. Use burdock root in stews, soups, and broths and in vinegars.

for a strong remedy), then pour into your mug. If using fresh herbs, either strain the infused milk into a mug or blend the herbs and milk thoroughly in a blender and then pour into a mug. Allow to cool to a comfortable drinking temperature. Stir in ¼ teaspoon of honey, if desired, and enjoy. Plan to consume the milk at once, and do not keep any that is left over.

A note on powdered herbs: If you purchase dried herbs or if you grow your own and dry them, use a grinder or blender to create a powder, then sift through a fine-mesh sieve and discard any large pieces. Alternatively, purchase powdered herbs (see Resources on page 232), and use a small whisk.

Sleep-Easy Hot Milk 1

 calming | YIELDS 1½ TEASPOONS POWDER BLEND,
PLUS 1 CUP HERBAL MILK (TWO ½-CUP SERVINGS)

For insomnia or feelings of fear, overwork, mental exhaustion, and worry that are keeping you from sleeping, this remedy is ideal. It combines the healing nature of sedative herbs with the tonic, relaxing properties of scalded milk, and on top of that, it is delicious. Prepare a mug of this hot milk an hour before bedtime and sip on it until ready for bed. A touch of maple syrup or chopped dates makes it a delicious treat anytime.

FOR THE SLEEP-EASY POWDER BLEND

½ teaspoon passionflower powder

½ teaspoon skullcap powder

½ teaspoon chamomile powder

FOR THE HOT HERBAL MILK

1 cup fresh (preferably raw) cow's milk or alternative milk of choice

½ teaspoon Sleep-Easy Powder Blend

1 date, chopped, or 3 to 5 drops pure maple syrup, optional

1 to 2 drops vanilla extract, optional

To make the powder blend, stir together the herb powders in a small glass jar, then cap and label. Store on the countertop.

To make a hot herbal milk, pour the milk into a small saucepan over medium heat. Add the date, if using. Heat until the milk scalds, just below the boiling point, about 5 to 8 minutes. Remove the pan from the heat and whisk in ½ teaspoon of the powder blend and the maple syrup and/or vanilla, if using. Strain into 2 warmed mugs and serve hot.

Sleep-Easy Hot Milk 2

 calming | YIELDS 1 CUP (TWO ½-CUP SERVINGS)

This version uses fresh wild lettuce, a wildflower that grows in many areas of the United States and in various habitats: poor soil, garden beds, roadsides, and fields. Wild lettuce lends sedative qualities when it is heated, as herbalist Euell Gibbons discovered when he sautéed the leaves and achieved a much more sedative action than he had experienced from eating them raw. If you have trouble sleeping, harvest these leaves before bedtime so you can enjoy the fresh air before you drink this hot milk and go to bed.

1 cup fresh (preferably raw) cow's milk or alternative milk of choice

1 cup chopped fresh wild lettuce leaves and stalks

¼ cup fresh or dried chamomile flowers

Pour the milk into a small saucepan over medium heat. Add the wild lettuce and chamomile and whisk. Heat until the milk scalds, just below the boiling point, about 5 to 8 minutes. Remove the pan from the heat, sweeten if desired, and strain into 2 warmed mugs. Serve hot.

Ayurvedic Tonic Milk

 stress support | YIELDS 1½ TEASPOONS POWDER BLEND,
PLUS 1 CUP HERBAL MILK (TWO ½-CUP SERVINGS)

Steeping fruits, seeds, and flowers in almond and rice milks is a traditional Ayurvedic method for relieving illnesses and toning the body in general. This recipe is a general tonic for stress, anxiety, fear, and difficult digestion due to these emotions.

FOR THE AYURVEDIC TONIC POWDER BLEND

½ teaspoon ashwagandha powder

½ teaspoon shatavari powder

½ teaspoon ginseng or eleuthero (Siberian ginseng) powder

FOR THE HOT HERBAL MILK

1 cup fresh (preferably raw) cow's milk or alternative milk of choice

2 cardamom pods

3 rose petals

1 date, chopped, or ¼ teaspoon honey, brown rice syrup, or date syrup, optional

½ teaspoon Ayurvedic Tonic Powder Blend

To make the powder blend, stir together the herb powders in a small glass jar, then cap and label. Store on the countertop.

To make a hot herbal milk, pour the milk into a small saucepan over medium heat. Add the cardamom, rose petals, and date, if using. Heat until the milk scalds, just below the boiling point, about 5 to 8 minutes. Remove the pan from the heat and whisk in ½ teaspoon of the powder blend. Add the honey, if using, and strain into 2 warmed mugs. Serve hot.

Morning Brain Tonic Milk

 clarity & memory | YIELDS ABOUT ¼ CUP POWDER BLEND,
PLUS 1 CUP HERBAL MILK (TWO ½-CUP SERVINGS)

To get your teenagers going on a cold morning—or to prepare yourself for a productive and active day—enjoy this energizing morning drink that stimulates mental clarity. Best served hot, this milk has a strong flavor, but it can be sweetened with licorice powder or chopped dates, and it can even be turned into a hot cocoa for those who need the extra persuasion: simply increase the licorice or cocoa powder to achieve the desired flavor.

FOR THE MORNING BRAIN TONIC POWDER BLEND

1 tablespoon plus 1 teaspoon amla powder

2 teaspoons ashwagandha powder

1 tablespoon plus 1 teaspoon gotu kola powder

1 teaspoon astragalus powder

FOR THE HOT HERBAL MILK

1 cup fresh (preferably raw) cow's milk or alternative milk of choice

½ to 1 teaspoon Morning Brain Tonic Powder Blend

½ teaspoon honey, or 1 date, chopped, optional

1 to 2 drops vanilla extract

Pinch of licorice root powder or cocoa powder

Tiny pinch of salt

To make the powder blend, stir together the herb powders in a small glass jar, then cap and label. Store on the countertop.

To make a hot herbal milk, pour the milk into a small saucepan over medium heat. Add the date, if using. Heat until the milk scalds, just below the boiling point, about 5 to 8 minutes. Remove the pan from the heat and whisk in ½ to 1 teaspoon of the powder blend and the honey (if using), vanilla, licorice, and salt. Strain into 2 warmed mugs and serve hot.

PASSIONFLOWER

Passiflora incarnata

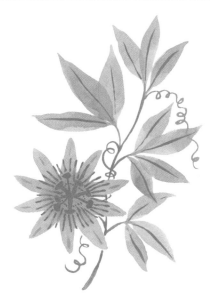

This lovely flower has long been used as a medicinal herb in the United States and Europe, Mexico, and Central America to ease insomnia, depression, and nervous debility. The flowers, leaves, and roots possess both stimulating alkaloids and sedative principles, which confounds researchers trying to determine how the herb works: specifically, it contains alkaloids, coumarins, phytosterols, and cyanogenic glycosides, among other potent phytochemicals. Generally, it is used as a sedative and to ease the body's response to chronic stress. It is contraindicated during pregnancy. Use passionflower in teas, infusions, syrups, honeys, and herb powder blends.

SKULLCAP

Scutellaria baicalensis (Chinese skullcap) and *S. lateriflora* (American skullcap)

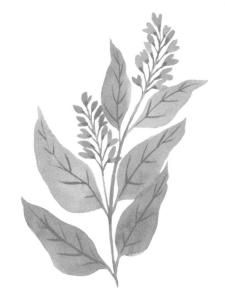

So named possibly because the flower resembles a cap on a head, skullcap has long been considered a nervine tonic and a mild sedative. This unassuming plant may help those suffering with stress, anxiety, headache, insomnia, and nervous tension, generally taken as a tea, capsule, tincture, or powder. Generally, American skullcap leaf acts as a sedative and nervine tonic, while Chinese skullcap root acts as an antispasmodic and anti-inflammatory, especially for headaches; it may also have some anticancer properties. Use either the root of Chinese skullcap or the leaf of American skullcap in teas, infusions, herb powder blends, honeys, and smoothie blends.

WILD LETTUCE

Lactuca canadensis and *L. scariola*

With their milky white, latex-like sap, wild lettuces inspired a great deal of plant symbolism in ancient Egyptian cultures, which appear to have valued lettuce both as a food and a fertility symbol. Pharaoh Hatshepsut possibly grew it in her gardens as a ritual herb because the white sap represented mother's milk, and it may have been used in birthing ceremonies, fertility rites, and nursing ceremonies.

For years in the United States, wild lettuce was listed as an official medicine in the *United States Pharmacopeia National Formulary*, and it was widely regarded as a gentle sleep aid, but its exceedingly mild qualities caused it to be dropped in 1916. Herbalists today sometimes combine it with valerian, roses, and other sedative herbs for children for a safe, gentle sleep inducer. In the 1960s, wild foods forager Euell Gibbons ate wild lettuce raw and found no soporific qualities but reported that, when he ate the greens stewed or steamed, he "became aware of a sort of languid drowsiness and feeling of well-being, as though I didn't have a care in the world." Young wild lettuce leaves can be chopped and added to stews and hot skillet dishes with salt and pepper. The taste is mild, and the texture is soft; a quick sauté in a hot pan is recommended.

Digestive Milk

 digestive support | YIELDS 1 CUP (TWO ½-CUP SERVINGS)

The flavor combination of fennel, fenugreek, and triphala is pleasant and a bit uplifting. It makes a soothing combination with hot milk, and is equally nice in hot apple cider.

- 1 cup fresh (preferably raw) cow's milk or alternative milk of choice
- ½ teaspoon Digestive Powder Blend (page 118)
- 1 date, chopped, optional

Pour the milk into a small saucepan over medium heat. Add the date, if using. Heat until the milk scalds, just below the boiling point, about 5 to 8 minutes. Remove the pan from the heat and whisk in ½ teaspoon of the powder blend. Strain into 2 warmed mugs and serve hot.

SHATAVARI

Asparagus racemosus

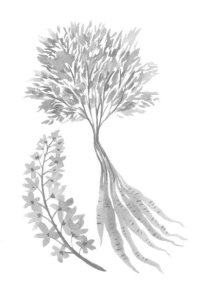

With the increasing demand for this and other medicinal herbs native to India, shatavari is being overharvested and may be endangered in its natural habitat. The root and stem have been used in Ayurvedic medicine to support women's health, and they contain plant chemicals similar to those in wild yams, including diosgenin. Shatavari has been used to soothe inflamed reproductive tissues and for infertility. Use the powder in smoothie blends and honeys, or prepare a tea with the dried roots.

GINSENG

Panax quinquefolius (American ginseng) and *P. ginseng* (Chinese or Korean ginseng)

The strongest ginseng is *Panax ginseng,* a plant native to Asia and used as a stimulating adaptogen, an herb that eases the way the body reacts to chronic stress. It originally grew in popularity as an energizing herb for men, providing vigor and endurance for a work day or during travel (it is considered yang: warming, energizing, and stimulant). It is now widely used for general exhaustion or insufficient energy within an organ or a system of organs, or as a tonic for debility. Ginseng is also being used with cancer patients undergoing chemotherapy and radiation.

The American species, *P. quinquefolius,* appears to have a more tonic action and is less stimulant. It is also used to warm, to invigorate, and to sustain, and Western herbalists tend to use it for men and women with fatigue, adrenal deficiency, and poor immune function. Ginseng's roots contain triterpenoid saponins, variously called ginsenosides and panaxosides, and are often used as a tonic for energy, drive, verve, focus, concentration, and all-around health.

Wild American ginseng is so overharvested that it is listed as an Appendix II plant on the federal Convention on International Trade in Endangered Species of Wild Fauna and Flora (CITES) List, meaning its commodity status is being closely watched because it may become threatened with extinction unless trade is controlled. Unfortunately, it is used in everything from true herbal medicine preparations to crackers, chips, and snacks.

Because of American ginseng's threatened status and the global overharvest of all ginsengs, I advocate using ginseng in a respectful and limited manner; it is useful in teas, decoctions, syrups, honeys, electuaries, herb powder blends, and broths.

Neither of these plants is to be confused with Siberian ginseng, *Eleutherococcus senticosus,* which is in the same family but different genus and has similar attributes.

Deep Sleep Milk

 calming | YIELDS ABOUT ¼ CUP POWDER BLEND, PLUS 1 CUP HERBAL MILK (TWO ½-CUP SERVINGS)

This blend is lovely, pleasant, and soothing. It's best taken in the evening to help achieve a peaceful, stress-free sleep.

FOR THE DEEP SLEEP POWDER BLEND

1 tablespoon plus 1 teaspoon shatavari powder

1 tablespoon plus 1 teaspoon ashwagandha powder

1 teaspoon fo-ti powder

1 teaspoon holy basil (tulsi) powder

FOR THE HOT HERBAL MILK

1 cup fresh (preferably raw) cow's milk or alternative milk of choice

½ teaspoon Deep Sleep Powder Blend

To make the powder blend, stir together the herb powders in a small glass jar, then cap and label. Store on the countertop.

To make a hot herbal milk, pour the milk into a small saucepan over medium heat. Heat until the milk scalds, just below the boiling point, about 5 to 8 minutes. Remove the pan from the heat and whisk in the powder blend. Pour into 2 warmed mugs and serve hot.

Hot or Chilled Lavender Milk

 calming | YIELDS 2 CUPS (FOUR ½-CUP SERVINGS)

Lavender milk is surprisingly versatile. Served hot, it can be just what's needed for the child who is scared of going to bed. It is soothing and relaxing and has a lovely light fragrance reminiscent of the garden. Served chilled, it can be a magical ingredient in a smoothie, or it can be enjoyed plain poured into tiny frosted glasses straight from the freezer on a hot day. It can be made with cream and whipped for a thick, luscious, flowery whipped cream (the perfect remedy for anxious children who can't relax), and made with whole milk, it is the basis for Lavender Yogurt (page 154). Rose petals can be substituted for the lavender for a similarly magical effect.

2 cups fresh (preferably raw) cow's milk or alternative milk of choice

2 cups fresh lavender flowers, or 1 cup dried

2 dates, chopped, or 2 teaspoons pure maple syrup, optional

In a medium saucepan over medium heat, combine the milk, lavender, and dates, if using. Heat until the milk scalds, just below the boiling point, about 5 to 8 minutes. Strain into a 1-quart jar (for cold milk) or 4 warmed mugs. Sweeten with maple syrup, if desired. Serve hot in the mugs, or allow the jar of herbal milk to come to room temperature (skimming off any skin that forms on top) and refrigerate to serve cold.

Spicy Rejuvenating Hot Licorice Milk

 energizing | YIELDS 2 CUPS (FOUR ½-CUP SERVINGS)

For those who like their hot milk with a little kick, this recipe will warm you up—and wake you up. These warming herbs and spices stimulate blood flow, ease congestion, and provide energy without caffeine. They are a delicious blend reminiscent of gingerbread, a perfect balance to the relaxing properties of hot milk. Sip a cup after a hard day at work or when you return from a brisk day of activities in a winter wonderland. Licorice is soothing on the throat and the tummy, and it gives the blend a natural sweetness.

FOR THE SPICY LICORICE BLEND

2 teaspoons ground ginger

1 teaspoon ground cinnamon

1 teaspoon licorice root powder

FOR THE HOT HERBAL MILK

2 cups fresh (preferably raw) cow's milk or alternative milk of choice

½ to 1 teaspoon Spicy Licorice Blend

2 cardamom pods

5 to 8 whole cloves

To make the powder blend, stir together the spices in a small glass jar, then cap and label. Store on the countertop.

To make the hot herbal milk, pour the milk into a small saucepan over medium heat. Add the Spicy Licorice Blend, cardamom, and cloves. Heat until the milk scalds, just below the boiling point, about 5 to 8 minutes. Strain out the solids and pour the milk into 4 hot mugs.

Gentle Tonic Milk for Building Strength

 nourishing | YIELDS 2 CUPS (FOUR ½-CUP SERVINGS)

If you're looking to improve your vigor and feel strengthened from the inside out, this nourishing drink will sustain you. Use fresh nettles, if possible, but dried nettles will work, too (just use one-third less). These herbs combine to provide minerals such as calcium and iron as well as energizing vitamins, and they create the scaffolding you need to build a healthy body. This tonic milk is thick, fragrant, and soothing on the throat.

    2 cups fresh packed nettle leaves

    2 cups fresh (preferably raw) cow's milk or alternative milk of choice

    1 teaspoon slippery elm powder

    1 teaspoon honey

Using gloves, hold the nettle stalks over a medium saucepan and use scissors to snip the leaves directly into the pan. Further snip them into small pieces in the pan. Pour the milk over the chopped leaves and place the pan over medium-low heat. Allow the nettle to steep in the heating milk, stirring frequently with a wire whisk to avoid scorching, until the milk is thick, dark green, and fragrant, about 10 to 15 minutes. Increase the heat to medium and continue to heat, stirring constantly, until the milk scalds, just below the boiling point. Remove the saucepan from the heat and allow the mixture to cool slightly. Whisk in the slippery elm powder and honey and strain into 4 warmed mugs. Drink hot.

FO-TI

Polygonum multiflorum

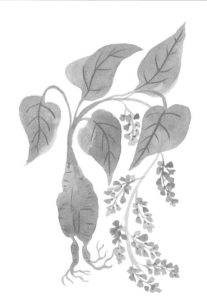

Historically used as a tonic in Traditional Chinese Medicine, the roots of fo-ti are used more as an energy herb than a medicine for physical ailments. Fo-ti has been valued for opening up energy channels in the body and restoring health, but taken long-term it can cause gastric upset. I find fo-ti's taste rather bland, which means it combines well with other energy and nervous-system-support herbs that have good flavor, such as licorice, red clover, wild sarsaparilla, and amla. Use the dried powder in smoothie blends and hot herbal milks, or steep the roots for tea.

SLIPPERY ELM

Ulmus rubra

One of the first herbs I learned about, slippery elms are trees native to North America. Their inner bark is carefully stripped from the branches and chopped or powdered for use, and I was first introduced to it as a food for convalescents. It is praised as a porridge and even as a tea, and although it is certainly nutritious, soothing, cooling, and mucilaginous, it is not very tasty. Perhaps its mildness is what makes it acceptable to someone who is sick and has no appetite. It does make a decent gruel when mixed with hot water or hot milk and sweetened with honey; otherwise, it can be added quite invisibly to smoothies and puddings, lending richness and creaminess thanks to its mucilage content.

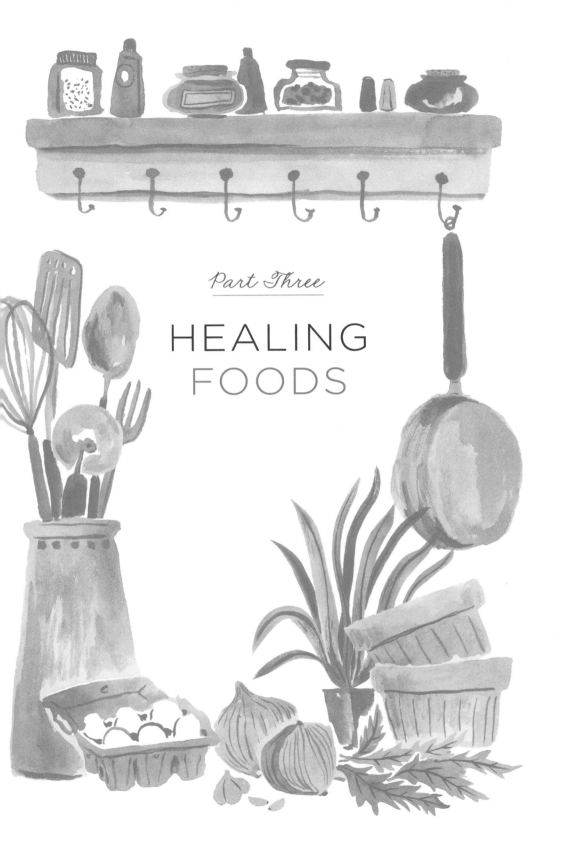

Part Three

HEALING
FOODS

9

NOURISHING BREAKFASTS

MORNING IS AN IDEAL TIME to use medicinal and healing herbs, as they are often high in nutrients, including minerals, vitamins, amino acids, and fiber, as well as flavor. Get creative with your breakfasts, enjoying herbs in traditional foods such as yogurt and cereals but also trying new morning foods, such as steamed greens and pickled vegetables. Together with protein-rich hard-boiled eggs, these foods provide the energy to begin a productive day.

Herbs can play a central part in all these types of foods: a bowl of steamed nettles with oil, vinegar, salt, and pepper is delicious in the morning, and a hearty bowl of cooked millet sprinkled with lamb's-quarter seeds or plantain seeds gives a satisfying crunch. Top with chopped avocado, nutritional yeast, chopped hard-boiled egg, or chopped tomato for a savory and filling breakfast—you won't miss the sweets.

In this chapter you'll find recipes for homemade yogurt, which is incredibly easy to make and fun to combine with various herbs for memorable flavors and aromas. You'll also find my family's favorite hot cereals, including a nut-and-seed granola (Iron-Rich Oat Granola, page 169), a summer muesli (Summer Morning Muesli with Fruit, page 161), and a hearty oatmeal (Hot Hearty Oatmeal, page 159). Each of these is an opportunity to nourish yourself with delicious herbs, including lavender and lemon balm, and with immune-supporting berries such as elderberry, blueberry, goji berry, and hawthorn berry. Experiment with fenugreek for its digestive benefits and with lemongrass for its stimulating aroma. Add herb powders, such as warming rhodiola powder, to your flour mixes (½ teaspoon per cup), or sprinkle calming ashwagandha powder into hot oatmeal. Serve with a mug of hot herbal tea (such as Mental Clari-Tea, page 86, or Heart-to-Heart Tea, page 91), and you'll have a delicious breakfast that nourishes the mind, the body, and the senses.

YOGURTS

A creamy treat and a healthy breakfast, yogurt is an ancient food honored for its simplicity as well as its beneficial effects on gut bacteria. If you love to eat a bowl of fresh, creamy yogurt with your breakfast, the following recipes will make your already-healthy yogurt even more flavorful and beneficial. The following recipes hint at the breadth of flavors that mix well with yogurt. Do your own experiments with various herbs; each will lend its own aroma, flavor, and sometimes even color (nettle produces a light green yogurt, for instance).

Also experiment with the types of milk you use, because different milks produce yogurts of varying thickness and texture. Dairy (cow and goat) milks produce the thickest and most reliable yogurt, but nut and seed milks can also be used; they will produce a thinner yogurt and may require the addition of thickening agents such as chia seeds, pectin, agar agar, arrowroot powder, or tapioca starch (see the Yogurt-Making Charts, page 153–54). The thinner yogurt produced with nut and grain milks can be used like buttermilk: for drinking and using in baking or smoothies. Dairy-based yogurt starters provide the most reliable results (use a few tablespoons of a previous batch of homemade yogurt or container of store-bought plain dairy yogurt). Nondairy yogurts and vegan yogurt starters are also available, but again, the resulting yogurt will be quite thin. Sweeten your yogurt with restraint: if you really want a bit of sweetness, avoid cane sugar and add honey or maple syrup upon serving, after the culturing process is complete.

Yogurt is versatile—it can be used in sauces, creams, soups, and smoothies—so it's easy to be creative with it, making it a wonderful way to include a variety of herbs, spices, and fruits in your diet. Depending on the herbs you choose, it can also help promote body strength and stamina.

How to Make an Herbal Yogurt

Although yogurt making is very simple, it requires a few special pieces of equipment. Fortunately, most kitchens already have them: a candy thermometer, a cooler (or a box with a thick blanket or several towels inside), and canning jars with lids. You'll also need a starter culture from a previous batch of plain, unsweetened yogurt (either homemade or store-bought). For dairy milks, use a dairy starter: for a thick yogurt, use a Greek-style yogurt as your starter; if you like it thinner, Dannon or Stonyfield brands will work. For almond milk, a dairy starter will work, or you can use a previous batch of almond yogurt, a package of vegan yogurt starter, or the contents of opened probiotic capsules, available at health food stores.

The process is simple—begin by heating the milk: Pour ½ gallon of milk into a medium stainless steel pot and place over high heat. Clip the candy thermometer onto the side of the pot, and have a whisk handy. Stir in any fresh or dried herbs called for in the recipe, and keep a careful eye on the milk as it heats on the stove, whisking frequently. When the thermometer reads exactly 180°F, remove the pot from the heat and allow it to cool, uncovered, until the temperature reads 114°F. This will take 1 hour or so.

Meanwhile, prepare your equipment: Retrieve a small cooler for your yogurt to culture in, and place a couple of towels or a blanket in it. Decide where you will place the cooler for the culturing period, and assemble several more blankets or coats at that location—I will sometimes put the cooler on my bed so I can easily wrap blankets around it and pop a pillow on top of it. (The yogurt thickens throughout the day, and when I'm ready for bed, I put the jars in the refrigerator. The yogurt is perfect in the morning.) After your space is prepared, turn your attention back to the milk. When the thermometer reads about 116°F, fill two 1-quart glass canning jars and a 1-pint glass canning jar with hot tap water and set them aside.

When the thermometer reads 114°F, empty the hot water from the glass jars and remove your starter culture from the refrigerator. If herbs have been added to the milk, strain them out and compost them. Add 2 to 3 tablespoons of starter and any powdered herbs to the milk and stir gently to incorporate. If using a sweetener, add it now, stirring well. Pour the cultured milk into the empty, warm 1-quart jars (I find using a ladle is less messy) and fill to the top; if there is extra milk, pour it into the pint jar. I've found that adding a little drizzle (about ½ teaspoon) of starter to the top of each filled jar helps the yogurt set better. Cap the jars and gently tuck them into the towels or blanket inside the cooler.

Carry the cooler to a place where it can sit for the next 4 to 12 hours, and cover the whole thing with a thick or woolen blanket, coats, pillows—anything that will help insulate the cooler. The milk needs to stay warm so that the bacteria can grow; this is what "sets" the milk and turns it into yogurt. After 4 hours, check the yogurt to see if it has set. With the lid still on the jar, turn the jar and watch the top half inch. The yogurt should appear solid. If you notice liquid or much movement, it is not set yet. If it has not set yet, place it back in the cooler for up to 8 more hours. (I often have the best results when I allow my yogurt to set overnight.) You can also drizzle another teaspoon of starter on top after 4 hours.

Once set, transfer the jars to the refrigerator. Use dairy yogurts within 2 weeks, and use nut or vegan yogurts within 2 days.

Yogurt-Making Charts

On the following pages, various dairy and alternative milks are compared as yogurt-making ingredients—first, using a dairy yogurt starter and second, using an almond yogurt starter and, in some cases, a thickener such as pectin or tapioca. Many vegan "yogurts" are so thin they can't be eaten with a spoon and should be used in smoothies or as a buttermilk substitute in baking. Use these charts to determine which milk and thickener will yield the texture and flavor you prefer.

YOGURT-MAKING CHART USING DAIRY STARTER

MILK	STRAIN?	TEXTURE	TASTE
ALMOND	No	Runny; results in curds and whey (lots of whey)	Sweet and tangy, very good
COCONUT	A little	Thick	Tart
DAIRY Dannon starter	No	Medium-thick, creamy	Tart and tangy
DAIRY Chobani starter	No	Very thick	Tart and tangy
HEMP	No, use like buttermilk	Very creamy	Slightly sweet, pleasantly tart
OAT	No, use like buttermilk	Thin	Very sweet, slightly tart
QUINOA	No, use like buttermilk	Extremely runny	Very tart, unpleasant
RICE	No	Thin	Tangy and pleasant
SOY	Very little	Thick	Pleasant

YOGURT-MAKING CHART USING **ALMOND STARTER**

MILK	THICKENER	STRAIN?	TEXTURE	TASTE
ALMOND	Pectin	No, shake and use like buttermilk	Very thin	Sweet, very good
COCONUT	Pectin	No, shake and use like buttermilk	Very runny	Slightly tart
HEMP	Tapioca	No, use like buttermilk	Thick, bubbly	Yeasty, like beer; strong flavor
OAT	Tapioca	No, use like buttermilk	Thin	Slightly sweet, pleasantly tart
QUINOA		No, use like buttermilk	Extremely runny	Very tart, unpleasant
SOY		Very little	Thin	Lightly sweet, tangy

Lavender Yogurt

 stress support | YIELDS 2 QUARTS

This yogurt lets the herbs' delicate flavors and aromas shine through. With the calming accent of lavender, it is lovely on pancakes or cardamom bread or dolloped onto lavender or rose-water scones.

> 2 quarts milk (dairy, oat, or soy is best)
>
> 1 cup fresh lavender flowers and/or leaves, or 2 cups dried
>
> 2 tablespoons starter culture

Pour the milk into a medium pot and add the lavender. Prepare the equipment and follow the instructions in "How to Make an Herbal Yogurt" (page 151).

LAVENDER

Lavandula angustifolia

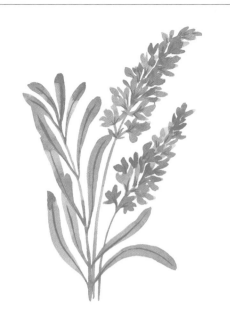

Renowned for its soothing effects, lavender's scent is therapeutic, sedating, and calming to the nervous system. However, lavender essential oil can be stimulating. The essential oil is antibacterial and antiseptic and reduces scar tissue formation when applied to fresh burns; it is often used in toiletries such as bath salts, perfume, and soaps. Fresh or dried lavender leaves and flowers can be a welcome addition to teas, infusions, syrups, honeys, electuaries, herb powder blends, herbal milks, and yogurts.

Citrus Yogurt

 refreshing | YIELDS 2 QUARTS

A bright, enchanting citrus-flavored yogurt, this is perfect on granola, in smoothies, on slices of orange, or drizzled onto lemon pound cake.

- 2 quarts milk (cow, goat, or almond is best)
- 1 cup chopped fresh orange and/or lemon peel, or 2 cups dried
- ¼ cup chopped fresh herbs (such as lemon balm, lemongrass, and/or lemon verbena), or 2 tablespoons dried
- 1 teaspoon lemon peel powder or lemon zest powder, optional
- 2 tablespoons starter culture

Pour the milk into a medium pot and add the herbs and lemon peel. Prepare the equipment and follow the instructions in "How to Make an Herbal Yogurt" (page 151).

LEMON VERBENA

Aloysia citrodora

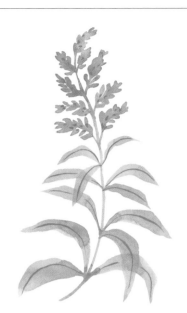

The lemony-scented leaves of lemon verbena have long been used in culinary traditions throughout Europe and North America for flavoring vegetables, salads, beverages, and desserts. Popular as an herbal tea, lemon verbena should not be confused with vervain (*Verbena hastata* or *V. officinalis*), which is a different plant entirely and lacks a lemony flavor.

LEMON BALM

Melissa officinalis

A medicinal powerhouse, *Melissa* (Greek for "bee") is affectionately called the "gladdening herb," due to our emotional response on smelling or ingesting the herb. It is rich in essential oils that reduce tension and relax the nervous system and at the same time heighten mental clarity. It is valued for promoting better memory and is a favorite of test-taking students. Some herbalists use lemon balm leaves to support kids and adults with ADD/ADHD, and many use it as a carminative, an aromatic herb that helps ease upset tummies, digestive spasms, and chronic and acute gas. Lemon balm can be safely used long-term as a nervine tonic, and it combines well with other herbs for a tea or infusion; it is delicious and helpful in vinegars and syrups, and the dried leaves can be powdered for smoothies. The fresh leaves can be nibbled but are not the best salad herbs because they tend to be mealy and fibrous; however, they are excellent extracted into water, vinegar, or honey.

Tropical Coconut and Cardamom Yogurt

 refreshing | YIELDS 2 QUARTS

This creamy yogurt can be used a key ingredient in spicy Indian cooking, or sweetener can be added to create a sweet enchanting treat. Let your nose be your guide when adding the cardamom: start with a little and add more until it smells as strong as you want it to taste.

2 quarts fresh (preferably raw) cow's milk, or alternative milk of choice

1 cup shredded coconut

1 teaspoon ground cardamom

2 tablespoons starter culture

Pour the milk into a medium pot and add the coconut. Prepare the equipment and follow the instructions in "How to Make an Herbal Yogurt" (page 151).

Maple Yogurt with Fenugreek

 digestive support | YIELDS 2 QUARTS

Fenugreek is traditionally used to support healthy digestion, ease bronchial spasms and coughing, and increase breast-milk production for nursing mothers. Naturally bitter, the seeds should be toasted in a dry pan for this recipe to reduce the bitterness and allow the sweetness to shine through. This is a sweet yogurt that is right at home on top of fresh, hot pancakes and waffles.

2 quarts fresh (preferably raw) cow's milk, or alternative milk of choice

½ cup fenugreek seeds, toasted in a hot, dry skillet

2 tablespoons starter culture

¼ cup pure maple syrup

Pour the milk into a medium pot and add the fenugreek. Prepare the equipment and follow the instructions in "How to Make an Herbal Yogurt" (page 151). (Strain out the seeds before adding the starter culture.)

FENUGREEK

Trigonella foenum-graecum

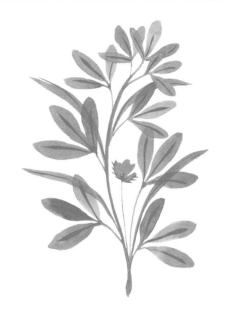

An ancient remedy for respiratory distress, bronchitis, pneumonia, and asthma, fenugreek is still relied on today for its expectorant properties in respiratory illness. Used primarily topically in the past, for sores, gout, and skin wounds, today fenugreek is commonly used to relieve respiratory and digestive complaints and to help increase the flow of breast milk in nursing mothers—aromatic fenugreek stimulates milk secretion and also eases the baby's colic. It is generally recognized as safe by the FDA and is widely considered to be a food or spice. It often gives the urine and sweat (and breast milk) the scent (or flavor) of maple syrup. Herbalist Aviva Romm advises caution for those with diabetes or hypoglycemia, as fenugreek seed in large quantities may slightly lower blood glucose levels. Avoid if pregnant. Enjoy fenugreek seeds in teas and decoctions, mulling blends, honeys, elixirs, vinegars, herbal milks, puddings, and yogurts, keeping in mind the sweet scent comes through as a mildly bitter flavor.

GRAIN-BASED BREAKFASTS

Create these hearty nut-, seed-, and herb-rich breakfasts for a strong start to your day. My family loves these delicious and nourishing breakfast staples according to the season: hot oatmeal with seeds and nuts throughout the winter, and muesli and granola with fruit in the summer. These recipes are versatile, so feel free to substitute other ingredients and use what grows near you.

Oats are the wonder seeds of *Avena sativa*, a very nourishing herb and food high in soluble fiber that lowers cholesterol. Eating protein-rich oats gives a feeling of fullness, protects the heart, and strengthens the bones, hair, and skin with its high calcium content. Its mild flavor lets other ingredients shine through.

CHIA

Salvia hispanica

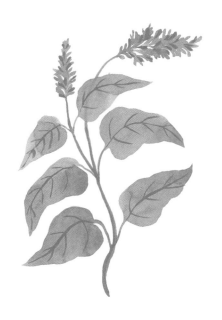

I love that the plant that produces this nutritious seed is blessed with the name *Salvia*. It is native to central and southern Mexico and Guatemala, where chia seeds used to be a staple crop. Chia seeds are growing in popularity as a food and supplement in the United States. People enjoy that they swell in size when steeped in water, creating a glutinous texture that is useful in drinks, breads, and custards. Chia seeds are very high in dietary fiber, protein, calcium, and other minerals, making them a valuable nutrient resource, especially because they can be eaten raw, with their vitamins and enzymes intact. They can also be cooked, so experiment with chia in soups, stews, breads, puddings, and granolas.

Hot Hearty Oatmeal

 heart support   *stress support* | YIELDS 1 CUP

Formerly called porridge, this is the thick breakfast cereal that, when cooked properly, becomes a delicious and satisfying morning staple. Experiment with all sorts of additions—nuts, seeds, milk, sweeteners, dried fruit, fresh fruit, and herb powders—and make this healthy meal every morning.

½ **cup rolled oats**

1 **cup water**

Additions—choose from the following:

2 **tablespoons sunflower seeds or flaxseeds**

1 **to 2 tablespoons chopped almonds or walnuts**

¼ **cup dried raisins, cranberries, or cherries**

1 **tablespoon dried plantain seeds or lamb's-quarter seeds**

¼ **cup shredded coconut**

1 teaspoon chia seeds

1 teaspoon herb powder (ground cinnamon, ashwagandha powder, or any of the blends on pages 115-42

1 teaspoon milk, butter, coconut oil, or flaxseed oil

Chopped fresh grapes, peaches, plums, bananas, apples, or cherries

Combine the oats and water in a small saucepan over medium heat. Bring to a low boil, then reduce the heat to low and cook, stirring frequently, until the oatmeal thickens, about 8 to 10 minutes. Scrape into your favorite breakfast bowl, and stir in your additions of choice. Serve hot.

Savory Millet Breakfast Bowl

YIELDS 1 TO 1½ CUPS

For those wishing to avoid oats, millet makes a hearty and wholesome substitute. You can cook whole millet for a loose and grainy dish resembling rice pilaf or grind the millet seeds first to achieve a creamy texture similar to polenta or grits, as in this recipe. The grain is slightly bitter, so sweeten if desired, or follow this recipe for a savory and fulfilling breakfast meal.

⅓ cup uncooked millet

¾ cup water

½ avocado, chopped

1 teaspoon nutritional yeast flakes

½ cup chopped tomatoes

Pinch of salt

In a blender, blend the millet into a coarse powder. Combine the millet and water in a small saucepan over high heat. Bring to a boil, then reduce the heat to low and simmer, stirring frequently, until the millet reaches a thick, porridge consistency, about 10 minutes. Scrape into a bowl and stir in the avocado, nutritional yeast, tomatoes, and salt. Enjoy hot.

Summer Morning Muesli with Fruit

 heart support | YIELDS TWO 1-CUP SERVINGS

Quick and simple to prepare, this is a satisfying breakfast packed with nutrients. It requires no cooking: just combine the ingredients in a bowl and enjoy! For a creamy muesli, combine the oats with the yogurt the night before, or if you like a bit more tooth, put it all together in the morning right before eating it. High in fiber, the plantain and lamb's-quarter seeds add a pleasant crunch.

> 1 cup rolled oats
>
> 1 cup yogurt (see page 151 for how to make your own)
>
> Additions—choose from several of the following:
>
>> 2 tablespoons sunflower seeds or flaxseeds
>>
>> 1 to 2 tablespoons chopped almonds or walnuts
>>
>> ¼ cup dried raisins, cranberries, or cherries
>>
>> 1 tablespoon dried plantain seeds or lamb's-quarter seeds
>>
>> ¼ cup shredded coconut
>>
>> 1 teaspoon herb powder (ground cinnamon, ashwagandha powder, or any of the blends on pages 115-42)
>>
>> Chopped fresh grapes, peaches, plums, bananas, apples, or cherries

In your favorite breakfast bowl, combine the oats and yogurt with all the additions you wish.

Iron-Rich Oat Granola

 heart support *iron-rich* | YIELDS ABOUT 1 GALLON

I've made this granola for years, and it's our family's favorite. It's easy to adapt using other ingredients, too, so if you want to add shredded coconuts, cashews, chopped almonds, pumpkin seeds, chocolate chips, or powdered herbs, you can: this recipe will easily handle anything your imagination can throw at it. It makes a big batch—you'll end up with about a gallon, or 15 or so cups of granola, enough to last a family a week or so.

We eat this in the morning with our homemade yogurt or with milk, or we snack on it throughout the day when we want something crunchy. The trick is to whisk the wet ingredients together first before combining them, all at once, with the dry ingredients. Keep the oven temperature low—don't be tempted to rush it, or you'll end up with burnt granola. Sip a cup of tea while the fragrant granola is baking. Store it in a large glass jar or plastic tub on the countertop or in the pantry, and enjoy it with fresh fruit.

I've found herb powders such as elderberry powder and dandelion root powder work well eaten with granola; it's best to wait to add these to your bowl along with the milk or yogurt just before eating. (I measure my oats with a large empty yogurt container, which holds 4 cups.)

12 cups rolled oats

2 cups raw nuts or large seeds—choose one or more of the following:

    Sunflower seeds

    Chopped almonds

    Cashews

½ cup small seeds—choose one or more of the following:

    Sesame seeds

    Millet

    Amaranth

    Dried plantain seeds

    Dried nigella seeds

    Chia seeds

1 cup mild oil, such as sunflower, safflower, or canola

½ to 1 cup pure maple syrup (according to how sweet you want your granola)

2 tablespoons water

2 cups additional ingredients—choose one or more of the following:

    Shredded coconut

    Raisins

    Chopped dates

    Chopped dried apricots

    Dried cranberries

Preheat the oven to 300°F and get out 3 baking sheets. In a large bowl, stir together the oats, nuts, and seeds. Run your fingers through the mix just for the pleasure of it, then set the bowl aside.

In a medium bowl, whisk together the oil, maple syrup, and water. Pour the liquid mixture into the oat mixture and stir to thoroughly combine. Pour the mixture onto the baking sheets and spread out into a thin layer.

Bake for 25 to 35 minutes, reaching in frequently to stir with a long wooden spoon, until golden and fragrant but not brown. (In our family, many of these "granola spoons" were carved by our son when he was 7 and 8 years old.) Be careful not to burn yourself! Remove the baking sheets from the oven, set them on wire racks or towels, and allow the granola to cool completely. Sprinkle with your additional ingredients of choice and stir together. Scrape the final mixture into a large glass jar or tub with a lid, and store at room temperature.

Berry Energy Balls

 energizing | YIELDS ABOUT 20 TO 25 ONE-INCH BALLS

These are tangy and delicious and give a bit of energy—both short-term energy and long-term staying power. Taste the mixture before rolling it into balls and adjust for flavoring. Great for a breakfast on the run, they can also be paired with a hard-boiled egg and steamed asparagus, broccoli, or carrots for an energizing morning meal.

1 cup sunflower seed butter

½ cup uncooked millet

¼ cup raw sunflower seeds

¼ cup flaxseeds

1 teaspoon elderberry powder

1 teaspoon Siberian ginseng powder or amla powder

¼ teaspoon ground ginger

¼ cup raisins

2 to 4 teaspoons pure maple syrup

½ teaspoon vanilla extract

¼ teaspoon ground cinnamon

Pinch of salt

2 to 4 teaspoons cocoa powder or carob powder, optional

In a medium bowl, stir together all the ingredients until well combined. Adjust for seasoning and for texture: add more millet and herb powder if the mixture is too gooey, or more maple syrup if it's too hard.

Put the cocoa powder into a small bowl, if using. Using your hands or two spoons, roll the mixture into 1-inch balls. Lightly roll the balls in cocoa powder, if desired. Layer the balls between sheets of wax paper in a dish with a snap-on lid. Refrigerate. Alternatively, spread out the mixture in a thin layer in a shallow glass dish and refrigerate; once chilled, slice into "bars" when you're ready to eat.

ELEUTHERO (SIBERIAN GINSENG)
Eleutherococcus senticosus

Appreciated as an adaptogen, the root of this plant is tonic for both men and women and is used to help alleviate feelings of stress, anxiety, and exhaustion. It protects against the chronic effects of the "fight-or-flight" hormones and reduces inflammatory responses, aids in relaxation, and boosts muscle and mental performance. Used as a tonic, this bland-tasting dried root can be used powdered, in smoothie blends and electuaries, or chopped in teas, infusions, decoctions, and syrups.

10

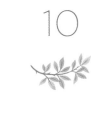

SNACKS

Instead of reaching for sweets as a mid-afternoon snack, or for corn chips that will leave you drowsy, make these simple snacks in advance so they're ready when you need a pick-me-up. These recipes allow fresh herbs to shine, such as chlorophyll-rich cilantro and parsley, and they use unusual herbs such as hyssop to introduce lovely and surprising flavors to your snack time.

Several of these recipes include high-protein foods, such as chickpeas, seeds, or cheese, to give you a substantial (and tasty) boost in the mid-afternoon.

SPREADS, DIPS, AND NUT BUTTERS

These delicious spreads, dips, and nut butters are similar to traditional recipes, but the addition of nutritious herbs makes them all the better. These are excellent eaten with chips, crackers, or rice cakes. Spread them on a warm slice of homemade bread, or cut up a platter of crisp carrots and bell peppers and serve them up together for a fresh snack.

Salsa Verde by Jan Buhrman

 energizing *immune support* | YIELDS ABOUT 9 CUPS

Internationally known chef and caterer Jan Buhrman shares her favorite salsa recipe using the freshest herbs of the garden. "This is one of those sleeper salsas that everyone wants the recipe for," she says, adding that the flavor secret is the anchovies. "Anchovies are about the best fish you can eat for the biggest bang for your buck." She's packed this salsa with heart-healthy garlic and fresh green herbs such as cilantro, chives, oregano, and even sage. The main ingredient, parsley, is traditionally used to stimulate the appetite, improve digestion, and assist with the healing of urinary tract infections. Because it can stimulate uterine contractions, pregnant women should omit the parsley and substitute lamb's-quarters or spinach.

2 garlic cloves

6 anchovy filets

3 cups chopped fresh Italian flat-leaf parsley

2 cups chopped fresh chives

1 cup chopped fresh oregano

½ cup chopped fresh sage

1 cup chopped fresh cilantro

¼ cup capers, rinsed and chopped

2 cups extra-virgin olive oil

¼ cup red wine vinegar

Zest of 1 lemon

1 cup minced shallots

Salt and ground black pepper, to taste

Using a mortar and pestle, crush the garlic and anchovies together to create a fine paste. Scrape into a large bowl. Add the parsley, chives, oregano, sage, cilantro, capers, olive oil, vinegar, lemon zest, and shallots (see note) and stir until well incorporated. Season with salt and pepper to taste. Transfer to an airtight container and store in the refrigerator for up to 1 week.

NOTE: If planning to freeze the salsa for later use, do not add the shallots at this stage. Place the salsa in a freezer-safe storage container, cover with a layer of olive oil, and freeze for up to 1 week. To serve, thaw and stir in the shallots.

PARSLEY

Petroselinum crispum

Common garden parsley is a nutrient powerhouse. Its pungent taste belies a bevy of minerals and vitamins, including folic acid, beta-carotene, flavonoids, and antioxidants. It tastes strong and bitter and is a warming circulatory stimulant, and best avoided by pregnant women. Nursing women should also avoid it because it is astringent and can decrease breast-milk production. As a food, parsley is enjoyed worldwide with meats and fish and in salads, condiments, and more. Eat parsley raw, chop it into your salads, and certainly infuse your vinegar with it. Also try it with your sautéed nettles and in your bone broths. Infuse olive oil with fresh parsley and garlic scapes, or chop it into honey that you plan to mix with vinegar for an elixir.

Minty Tahini with Hyssop

 nourishing | YIELDS 1 CUP

A simple sesame tahini can be made into a digestive helper when blended with a carminative herb such as mint, dill, or anise hyssop. A little goes a long way in this recipe, so don't overdo it: let your nose be your guide, and taste it throughout the process.

1 cup raw sesame seeds

2 to 4 tablespoons crumbled dried mint or anise hyssop leaves

Salt, to taste

2 tablespoons extra-virgin olive oil, if needed

In a heavy skillet over medium heat, toast the sesame seeds until fragrant, about 5 minutes. Add the mint and cook, stirring continuously, for 1 minute. Add the salt and cook for 1 minute more. Transfer the mixture onto a plate and allow to cool. When cool, puree the mixture in a blender or food processor until creamy. Add olive oil, if needed, to achieve the consistency you desire. Store in the refrigerator for up to 5 days.

Hummus with Parsley

I love making chickpea hummus because it has such a depth of flavor and is full of iron and protein. Traditionally, Middle Eastern recipes for hummus, or *hummus bi tahini*, are spicy, thin, drizzled with a great deal of olive oil, and sprinkled with paprika. This hummus is a variation that incorporates the sharp flavor of parsley. A powerhouse of minerals, one cup of fresh, raw parsley provides 83 mg of calcium, 332 mg of potassium, and almost 80 mg of vitamin C. It's extremely high in vitamins A and K. Use this as a dip with carrots, red bell peppers, crackers, or rice cakes.

3 cups cooked chickpeas

½ cup tahini (sesame paste, such as Minty Tahini with Hyssop, page 167), optional

½ cup warm water

1 cup chopped fresh parsley, or 3 tablespoons dried

1 teaspoon garlic powder

½ cup lemon juice

1 to 2 cups extra-virgin olive oil

1 to 2 teaspoons salt

Pinch of paprika, for garnish

In a blender or food processor, puree the chickpeas, tahini (if using), water, parsley, garlic powder, and lemon juice. Blend until coarsely ground. With the motor running, add the olive oil until the desired consistency is reached, remembering that the hummus will thicken as it sits. Add the salt a little at a time, according to taste. Transfer to a shallow bowl and serve drizzled with extra olive oil and sprinkled with paprika.

Nettle Cream Cheese Dip

This is a great dip to make with the nettle leaves left over from making tea or an infusion. Don't just compost them! Brew your tea and strain it, drinking the liquid and reserving the leaves to use in this creamy dip. Of course, you can always chop fresh leaves to use instead; they are soft and

puree easily. Mixed with cream cheese and some herbs for seasoning, nettles make a quick, nutritious dip.

> 1 to 2 cups chopped nettle leaves (reserved from making tea, freshly cooked, or fresh)
>
> 1 teaspoon minced fresh chives, parsley, or summer or winter savory
>
> ½ to 1 cup cream cheese
>
> Salt and ground black pepper, to taste

In a blender or food processor, puree the nettles and chives. Add the cream cheese a little at a time until the desired consistency is reached. Add salt and pepper to taste, and transfer to a small bowl to serve. Cover any leftovers and store in the refrigerator for up to 3 days.

Sunflower Spread with Chia Seeds

 nourishing | YIELDS ABOUT 1 CUP

This decadent "butter" has a heady, robust fragrance and a deep, nutty flavor. It's much earthier than raw peanut or almond butter, because toasting the seeds brings out a richness not found in raw seeds. Spread this on hot toast or rice cakes and top with a strong honey, such as Deep Forest Honey (page 55) or buckwheat honey, or top with slivered strawberries or fresh plum slices. Thin the recipe with a ¼ cup more oil to use as a dip with carrots or chips.

> 1 cup raw sunflower seeds
>
> 1 tablespoon chia seeds
>
> 1 tablespoon raw nigella seeds, optional
>
> 2 tablespoons olive or sunflower oil
>
> Pinch of salt, optional

In a heavy skillet over medium heat, lightly toast the sunflower seeds, stirring constantly, for 1 minute. Add the chia seeds and the nigella seeds, if desired, and toast for 1 more minute. Transfer the mixture onto a plate and allow to cool. When cool, pour the seed mixture into a blender or food processor, add the oil and the salt, if desired, and blend until creamy. Transfer to a ½-pint glass jar and store in the refrigerator for up to 2 weeks.

NIGELLA

Nigella sativa

These flowers are startlingly beautiful because they look like tiny, bright blue or white stars in the garden. After flowering, seed pouches form that contain very tiny black seeds, giving the plant its common names "black cumin" and "black caraway." Nigella is an ancient herb with folklore and archaeological evidence going back to Egyptian and biblical times; today it is used as a cooking spice, in confectionary, and in flatbreads such as naan. It gives a good crunch in granolas and breads, and can be sprinkled on oatmeal, mixed into crackers with flaxseed, or ground to be used as a powder.

Iron-Rich Pumpkin Seed Butter

 iron-rich | YIELDS ABOUT 1 CUP

Naturally high in iron, pumpkin seeds are also high in protein, calcium, potassium, and omega-6 and omega-9 essential fatty acids. Raw seeds have a mild taste, but toasting them brings out a rich, nutty flavor. Molasses is iron rich, and dandelion root is naturally high in iron and can be found powdered in health food stores. Spread this on toast or rice cakes for a robust flavor and boost of iron.

1 cup raw pumpkin seeds (pepitas)

2 tablespoons olive or sunflower oil

1 tablespoon dandelion root powder

Pinch of salt

1 teaspoon molasses or 1 date, pitted, optional

In a heavy skillet over medium heat, lightly toast the pumpkin seeds, stirring constantly, until fragrant, 2 to 3 minutes. Transfer onto a plate and allow to cool. When cool, pour the seeds into a blender or food processor and add the oil, dandelion root powder, salt, and molasses, if desired. Blend until creamy. Transfer to a ½-pint glass jar and store in the refrigerator for up to 2 weeks.

Herbal Cocoa Spread

 energizing | YIELDS ABOUT 2 CUPS

This is a rich, thick, and delicious spread that I love to put on rice cakes. It can be topped with jelly, honey, or slices of fresh plums or strawberries for a decadent yet nourishing treat.

2 cups roasted almond butter

2 to 4 tablespoons cocoa powder

2 tablespoons astragalus, ashwagandha, or amla powder, or a mix

¼ cup chocolate chips

1 tablespoon honey

2 to 4 tablespoons walnut, sunflower, or safflower oil

Pinch of salt

In the blender or food processor, blend the almond butter, cocoa, astragalus powder, chocolate chips, and honey, adding the oil as needed to achieve the desired consistency. Transfer to a 1-pint glass jar and store in the refrigerator for up to 4 weeks.

NOTE: Because this spread is so thick, the chips may or may not grind completely when added with the rest of the ingredients. Therefore, depending on your blender's strength and speed, you may want to grind them completely in the blender first. I find that grinding the chocolate chips first (before adding the other ingredients) tends to creates a smoother spread, while adding them later results in a chunky spread. Both ways are delicious!

AMLA

Emblica officinalis

Tart and tasty, the fruit of this Indian tree is considered a wonderful "Rasayana" herb in the Ayurvedic tradition, meaning it is used to restore and rejuvenate. It is now widely regarded as an antioxidant and adaptogenic herb, as well. Like other adaptogens, amla supports the mind and body against stress, and herbalist David Winston reports it supports connective tissue. Generally found as a powder in the West, amla is useful in powder blends, smoothies, honeys, electuaries, and hot herbal milks.

Cardamom Coconut Crème Dip by Blaire Edwards

 refreshing | YIELDS ABOUT 2 CUPS

"Outside of learning about plants, potlucks are the best part of attending herb school," says Florida herbalist Blaire Edwards. "Here is a refreshing dip I made and shared with my classmates during the wintertime—it pairs well with Gala apples, clementines, and pineapple chunks." Blaire sometimes ladles this dip on top of chocolate-and-espresso-bean crust and chills it in the refrigerator to make rich mini-pies. Plan ahead to soak the cashews in water for 2 hours before beginning the recipe.

1 cup cashews

2 tablespoons coconut oil

2 tablespoons coconut milk

¼ cup pure maple syrup

1 tablespoon vanilla extract

1½ teaspoons lemon juice

⅛ teaspoon salt

½ cup coconut yogurt or any yogurt

1 teaspoon ground cardamom

Put the cashews in a small bowl, cover with water, and allow to soak for at least 2 hours. Drain and rinse. (Soaking makes the cashews easier to puree and gets rid of anti-nutrients such as phytic acid.)

Melt the coconut oil in a small saucepan over the lowest possible heat. Set aside.

In a blender, blend the soaked cashews, coconut milk, maple syrup, vanilla, and lemon juice until smooth. With the blender running, add the melted coconut oil and salt. Pulse or stir in the coconut yogurt and cardamom. Adjust the sweetness and cardamom flavor to your liking, then scrape the crème into a bowl and serve.

SAVORY SNACKS

Home-baked breads and crackers are a fantastic place to use all those wild seeds from the garden and field: plantain, nigella, and lamb's-quarter seeds are plentiful in late summer and fall, and they provide a wonderful crunch and an abundance of fiber to our baked goods. Plantain puts its seeds on tall, obvious spikes, right off the ground and close together for easy picking; lamb's-quarter creates a mini-tree from which you can harvest a basketful of nutty-tasting seeds from just one plant.

Wheat and Wild Seed Peasant Bread

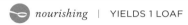 *nourishing* | YIELDS 1 LOAF

This is a recipe I've adapted from my bread machine's cookbook, specifically to include wild plant materials and to make the bread tastier and healthier. Some of my friends laugh when I tell them I use a bread machine, but it is actually a great time-saver and produces delicious results. If you don't have a bread machine, simply incorporate the ingredients into your favorite whole wheat sandwich bread recipe. For this bread-machine recipe, leave the seeds whole to add to the hearty texture of the peasant bread. This bread will be dense and hearty; enjoy it with butter (such as Sage Butter, page 48), honey (such as Angelica Honey for Digestion, page 58), or the Spicy Ginger Electuary on page 61. It's also delicious spread with a thick layer of Sunflower Spread with Chia Seeds (page 169) or Iron-Rich Pumpkin Seed Butter (page 170) and topped with thin slices of plum.

1½ cups water

2 cups whole wheat flour

2¼ cups bread flour

½ cup plantain seeds or lamb's-quarter seeds

¼ cup ground flaxseeds (you can also use amaranth seeds, chia, or millet)

2½ tablespoons butter

1½ teaspoons salt

2 teaspoons active dry yeast

Every bread machine is a bit different, so follow the directions for your machine. Add the ingredients in layers in the order listed. Run on the "whole wheat" setting, about 3½ hours. Turn the baked bread out onto a wire rack to cool completely before slicing.

PLANTAIN

Plantago major and *P. lanceolata*

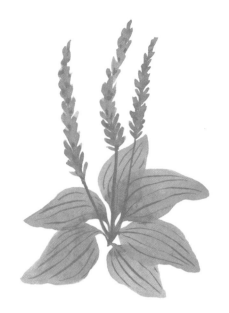

As a food source, plantain is most available in the early spring and fall. In the spring, look for its small, soft, succulent leaves as they sprout from the ground. Containing mucilage, glycosides, and silicic acid, these tender leaves make a decent addition to salads and may be steamed and sprinkled with vinegar. The fiber-rich seeds emerge in the fall at the top of a long stalk; when ripe, they can be harvested and used for food. Collect a basketful of seeds, lightly dry them on a screen, and store them in a tin. Sprinkle the seeds on oatmeal or include with wheat flour when baking bread; they add calcium, iron, and potassium.

All plantago seeds are laxative in large doses and form the basis for many over-the-counter preparations that list "psyllium" seeds, a related species. They work by forming a bulky, mucilaginous mass in the gut that stimulates peristalsis and pushes food material through the intestines. They are an excellent fiber/laxative combination that works in perfect harmony with lots of water.

Plantain leaves are also mucilaginous, making a pulpy mass when chewed and swallowed, which helps soothe the digestive tract and ease ulcers or burning. This makes them useful in hot herbal milks and even in medicinal stews or broths.

Golden Seed Crackers

These are truly delicious crackers! Bright yellow, thanks to the turmeric, and crunchy, these crackers are not bitter at all and, in fact, possess a depth of flavor not typically found in crackers. They are delicious on their own—savory, slightly salty, and flavorful—and are even better paired with a dip, such as Hummus with Parsley (page 168) or Nettle Cream Cheese Dip (page 168).

½ cup raw sunflower seeds

½ cup raw pumpkin seeds (pepitas)

½ cup chia seeds

½ cup other seeds, such as plantain, lamb's-quarter, nettle, or flax

1 rounded tablespoon ground turmeric

1 teaspoon plus a pinch of salt

1 cup water

Preheat the oven to 350°F. Line a baking sheet with parchment paper.

In a medium bowl, stir together the sunflower seeds, pumpkin seeds, chia seeds, and other seeds and the turmeric and 1 teaspoon of the salt until well combined. Add the water, stir well, and set aside for 10 minutes. This will allow the chia to gel.

Using a rubber spatula, spread the mixture evenly over the prepared baking sheet, spreading it to all sides and corners. Your goal is to get it as thin as possible, preferably about ⅛ inch thick. Sprinkle a pinch of salt on top and gently press it in with the spatula. Bake for 30 minutes.

Remove the pan from the oven. Using a large knife or a pizza cutter, carefully score the cracker layer into squares, rectangles, or diamonds—whatever shape you like—but do not cut all the way through. Holding the parchment paper, flip the entire layer of fused crackers and parchment upside down onto the pan. Be careful not to burn yourself! Peel the parchment paper off the cracker in one large sheet, then return the upside-down cracker to the oven to cook the other side. Bake for another 20 to 30 minutes, until the cracker layer is crisp, checking periodically to make sure it doesn't burn.

Remove the pan from the oven and allow the cracker layer to cool completely. Once cool, break the crackers along the scoring lines and store in an airtight container on the countertop for up to 1 week.

Green Seed Crackers

 nourishing | YIELDS ABOUT FORTY 2-INCH CRACKERS

Made without grains, these are a wonderful, crispy seed cracker for highlighting your favorite hummus. The iron-rich nettle powder makes them a deep green color, and they are not overly spicy—a perfect vehicle for a tangy dip. Make them with a nettle infusion for a well-rounded nettle experience.

½ cup raw sunflower seeds

½ cup raw pumpkin seeds (pepitas)

½ cup chia seeds

½ cup other seeds, such as plantain, lamb's-quarter, nettle, or flax

1 rounded tablespoon nettle powder

1 teaspoon plus a pinch of salt

1 cup water or Basic Nettle Infusion (page 95)

Follow the instructions for Golden Seed Crackers, page 175.

Caraway Crackers

 digestive support | YIELDS ABOUT FORTY 1-INCH CRACKERS

Fragrant and flavorful, the caraway flavor really comes through in these crackers packed with digestive herbs. They make a nice evening nibble when you want something after dinner but don't want anything sweet. Dip them into hot tea to soften them a bit, or pair with your favorite hummus or pesto, such as Wild Lamb's-Quarter Pesto (page 43) or Spring Weed Pesto (page 44). Find chickpea flour (a dense, nutrient-rich flour made from garbanzo beans) at your local health food store or specialty market.

2 cups chickpea flour

2 tablespoons extra-virgin olive oil

1 teaspoon baking powder

1 teaspoon salt

1 rounded tablespoon caraway seeds

1 rounded tablespoon aniseeds

1 rounded tablespoon fennel seeds

½ cup water

Preheat the oven to 350°F. Line a baking sheet with parchment paper.

In a medium bowl, combine all the ingredients and stir until there are no lumps. Using a rubber spatula, spread the dough evenly over the prepared baking sheet. Cover with another layer of parchment paper, and use a rolling pin to roll the dough as thin as possible, preferably ⅛ inch thick. Remove the top layer of paper and bake for 20 minutes.

Remove the pan from the oven. Using a large knife or a pizza cutter, gently score the cracker layer into squares, rectangles, or diamonds—whatever shape you like—but do not cut all the way through. Holding the parchment paper, flip the entire layer of fused crackers and parchment upside down onto the pan. Be careful not to burn yourself! Peel the parchment paper off the cracker in one large sheet, then return the upside-down cracker to the oven to cook the other side. Bake for another 15 to 20 minutes, until the cracker layer is crisp, checking periodically to make sure it doesn't burn.

Remove the pan from the oven and allow the cracker layer to cool completely. Once cool, break the crackers along the scoring lines and store in an airtight container on the countertop for up to 1 week.

Golden Popcorn

 nourishing | YIELDS ABOUT 1 CUP POPCORN DUST,
PLUS 3 TO 4 CUPS FLAVORED POPPED CORN

My kids love to drizzle olive oil on their fresh, hot popcorn and then sprinkle it all with nutritional yeast; they love the deep buttery flavor. Adding a bit of dulse, garlic, and other herbs to this mix heightens the depth of flavor, gives it little green flecks, and makes the popcorn more interesting (not to mention a little healthier!).

FOR THE GOLDEN POPCORN DUST

1 cup nutritional yeast

1 tablespoon dried dulse flakes

1 teaspoon garlic granules

1 teaspoon finely shredded dried dandelion leaf

1 teaspoon finely shredded dried basil leaf

Salt and ground black pepper, to taste

FOR THE POPCORN

½ cup popping corn

1 to 2 tablespoons extra-virgin olive oil

To make the popcorn dust, stir together all the popcorn dust ingredients in a small bowl. Transfer to a 1-pint glass jar, cap, and label. Store on a pantry shelf until ready to use.

To make the popcorn, pop the corn kernels in an air popper or in a dry hot skillet with a lid. Or do as we did when we went camping under the redwood trees: Mold an 8-inch-wide "bowl" out of aluminum foil and crease the ends almost shut, leaving a small hole. Pour in the corn kernels, seal the ends completely, and place the bowl on the coals of a campfire. Regardless of the way you pop your popcorn, listen for the first sounds of popping and be ready to grab the skillet or bowl quickly. Shake continuously while the corn is popping, and when the popping slows down to once every five seconds or so, take it off the heat and pour the popcorn into a wide, shallow bowl.

Drizzle the olive oil onto the freshly popped popcorn, then sprinkle a few teaspoons of the Golden Dust over the popcorn and stir it in. Adjust the seasonings and serve.

11

SALADS

WILD SALADS ARE EASY TO CREATE, and they give you a feeling of freshness and vigor that can come only from ingesting vibrant living plants picked in the sunshine. I think wild herbs contain a certain energy that is lacking in hybridized plants, especially those grown in overcultivated soils and processed mechanically. These salads are chock-full of the juiciness we need in life, so experiment with what grows near you, and be creative!

Herbs such as watercress (spicy), oxalis (sour), purslane (crunchy), and hyssop (minty) make for great additions to the salad bowl. Combine them with your favorite lettuces and spinach leaves to create a delicious and unique salad that begs for pickled cauliflower, chopped carrots, discs of celery, and creamy chunks of goat cheese.

The raw crunch of garden greens and herbs provides that certain something that makes a salad such a satisfying meal. It's green, it's fresh, it's got crunch but also a softness about it. It can be rich and creamy, or it can be drizzled with an acidic dressing with a bite. Salads are an ideal way to enjoy the bounty of summer herbs. Harvested fresh from the garden or the fields, these leaves, flower petals, seeds, stalks, and even roots offer us their vitamins, minerals, and goodness.

By including cultivated or wild herbs in your salad, you're giving your body a boost of flavor and nutrition through micronutrients not generally found in lettuce. Romaine lettuce typically contains vitamin A, vitamin K, potassium, and other trace metals and minerals, but not the triterpenoids or flavonoids of gotu kola, nor the quercetin of watercress. These special herbs lend both their unique flavors and their micronutrients to make these salad combinations hearty and delicious.

Make these salads with the freshest leaves and flowers available. Be sure to wash all the salad leaves and herbs and spin them dry in a salad spinner. If you'll have to wait before eating your salad, store the undressed leaves loosely in a plastic bag or tub. Rip the leaves into bite-size pieces and experiment with including chopped fresh dandelion root alongside your chopped carrots and fresh purslane stalks alongside your celery. Use a basic dressing of 2 or 3 parts olive oil to 1 part infused vinegar (or plain apple cider vinegar, balsamic vinegar, red wine vinegar, or lemon juice) with a dash of salt and pepper.

Get creative with herbal garnishes: sprinkle the whole salad with an abundance of colorful herbs, including fresh red clover blossoms, calendula petals, nasturtium petals, fennel flowers or fronds, dill flowers, nigella flowers, borage flowers, violet flowers and young leaves, bee balm petals, and chives from the garden, and black locust flowers or elder flowers from the wild.

Summary Solstice Salad

 digestive support | MAKES 4 TO 6 SERVINGS

When my herb school is in full summer swing, I often ask my apprentices to gather leaves from the garden for our community lunch. My student Blaire used to love this part of the day and would be the first out the door with the salad bowl; she would return bearing a fragrant, colorful mound of hyssop, lamb's-quarter, dandelion, violet leaves and flowers, purslane, borage leaves and flowers, bee balm petals, mustard leaves, wood sorrel, and a few sprigs of arugula and butter lettuce from the garden. We'd pour on homemade garlic-scape-infused olive oil and fruit-and-herb-infused balsamic vinegar, sprinkle with a little locally harvested sea salt, and voilà: a feast fit for a queen.

FOR THE SALAD

1 large handful of arugula, lettuce, or spinach

2 large handfuls of mixed herbs—choose from the following:

Lamb's-quarter leaves

Hyssop leaves

Dandelion leaves (young)

Violet flowers

Violet leaves (young)

Bee balm petals

Parsley leaves

Mustard leaves (young)

Wood sorrel

FOR THE DRESSING

½ cup oil (such as Strong Garlic Oil, page 36, Light Fennel and Borage Flower Salad Oil, page 38, or Lemony Salad Oil, page 38)

¾ cup balsamic vinegar, red wine vinegar, or Fruit Vinegar for Salads (page 34)

Salt and ground black pepper, to taste

To make the salad, tear the arugula into bite-size shreds and place them in a large salad bowl. Add a combination of as many of the herbs as you wish.

Pour the oil and vinegar over the salad and toss. Add salt and pepper to taste and toss again. Serve immediately.

Mind Tonic Salad

 clarity & memory | MAKES ABOUT 4 SERVINGS

Just as coffee is used as a vitalizing drink to make our minds alert, so have certain herbs been used since antiquity to wake up the mind—and they do it without caffeine. Lemon balm, lemon verbena, gotu kola, and rosemary are all valued as mind tonics, and when used in the right proportions, they happen to make a delicious and healthy salad.

FOR THE SALAD

2 handfuls of lettuce or spinach

1 handful of fresh gotu kola leaves

1 handful of fresh lemon balm leaves (very young), chopped

½ handful of fresh lemon verbena leaves, chopped

FOR THE DRESSING

¼ cup fresh rosemary leaves, or 1 tablespoon dried

1 teaspoon prepared horseradish (from a jar)

1 cup yogurt or sour cream

¼ cup extra-virgin olive oil

Salt and ground black pepper, to taste

To make the salad, tear the lettuce into bite-size shreds and place them in a large salad bowl with the gotu kola, lemon balm, and lemon verbena.

To make the dressing, blend the rosemary, horseradish, yogurt, and olive oil in a blender or whisk in a small bowl or jar until smooth and creamy. Add salt and pepper to taste. Pour the dressing over the salad and toss. Enjoy immediately.

GOTU KOLA

Centella asiatica

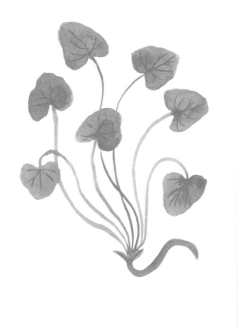

Also called *brahmi,* gotu kola is a small leafy plant that can easily be grown in a moist garden or streambed. It is traditionally used throughout Southeast Asia as a nervine tonic to stimulate mental clarity, cognitive function, and memory. The leaves are often paired with lemon balm, ginseng, ginkgo, rosemary, or motherwort for its gentle stimulation of the brain to think fast and remember. It is considered a nervine tonic for cases of insomnia and is a gentle vasodilator. Chew the mild-tasting young leaves fresh, enjoy them in salad, and use gotu kola in syrups, teas, honeys, sautés, herb powder blends, and chopped and added with chives to soft cheeses.

Fattoush Salad with Chickpeas and Feta

by Catherine Walthers

 nourishing | MAKES 6 SERVINGS

My Martha's Vineyard friend, a private chef, and the author of the *Soups and Sides* cookbook, Cathy Walthers shares this fresh and crunchy salad, which she describes as "along the lines of a Greek salad, only a bit better!" Cathy says,

> The word *fattoush* means "moistened bread," and the dish is of Syrian or Lebanese origin, combining the wonderful crunch of fresh vegetables and "croutons" with fresh herbs and the creaminess of sheep's milk feta cheese. It pairs well with a summer picnic sandwich or a bowl of soup, and it's easy to make: get creative and add chickpeas for additional protein.

FOR THE SALAD

Two 8-inch pita breads

1 tablespoon extra-virgin olive oil

1 head romaine lettuce or 2 romaine hearts, chopped into bite-size pieces

2 large cucumbers, peeled, seeded, and diced

½ red onion, very thinly sliced

2 cups cherry tomatoes, quartered

1 cup cooked chickpeas, drained and rinsed, optional

¼ cup minced fresh parsley

¼ cup shredded fresh mint

1 cup crumbled or diced feta cheese
(sheep's milk feta is wonderful)

FOR THE DRESSING

⅓ cup freshly squeezed lemon juice

⅓ cup extra-virgin olive oil

1 garlic clove, minced

1 teaspoon ground cumin

½ teaspoon kosher salt

Grind of black pepper

To make the salad, preheat the oven to 350°F. Completely separate the pita breads into two layers each and place them on a baking sheet. Brush each piece with the olive oil. Bake 8 to 10 minutes, until lightly crisp. Let the pitas cool, then break them into small, bite-size pieces like croutons and set aside.

In a large bowl or platter, combine the lettuce, cucumbers, onion, tomatoes, chickpeas (if using), parsley, and mint.

To make the dressing, whisk together all the dressing ingredients in a small bowl or jar. Just before serving, whisk the dressing again, pour over the salad, and toss. Toss in the toasted pita and top with the feta cheese.

Red Cabbage and Arame Salad by Brittany Nickerson

 iron-rich | MAKES FOUR 1-CUP SERVINGS

Arame is a type of seaweed found in temperate Pacific Ocean waters and is a favorite ingredient of practicing herbalist, health educator, and cook Brittany Nickerson. Brittany runs Thyme Herbal in Amherst, Massachusetts, and she shares that arame has a mild, pleasant taste and is tender enough to eat after soaking only, lending itself well to this salad. Brittany says,

> Loaded with vitamins and minerals, arame is particularly high in calcium, magnesium, iodine, iron, and vitamin A. Arame also has a high lignan content, a plant-based compound with antioxidant and anti-inflammatory actions in the body. Pacific arame is square and very thin, usually breaking into pieces about ½ to 1 inch in length after drying.

Combined with other rich Asian-inspired condiments, this colorful salad makes a great side dish or first course and can be served alongside almost anything. It can be completely prepared and dressed ahead of time and refrigerated until time to serve.

½ cup Pacific arame seaweed

⅓ cup toasted sesame seeds

1 small red cabbage

2 tablespoons tamari or soy sauce

2 tablespoons sugar-free rice wine vinegar

3 tablespoons sesame oil

In a small bowl, soak the arame in enough water to cover by 2 inches. Let sit for 5 minutes, then drain.

While the arame is draining, toast the sesame seeds in a heavy pan or cast iron skillet over low heat, stirring frequently so they do not burn. Once the seeds begin to turn golden brown they are ready, about 5 to 10 minutes. Set aside.

Cut the cabbage into quarters and remove the core. Thinly slice the cabbage into ¼- by 2-inch slices to yield about 4 cups of slices. Toss the cabbage slices in a large salad bowl with the drained arame. Add the toasted sesame seeds, tamari, rice wine vinegar, and sesame oil, and toss well.

Spicy Watercress Salad with Creamy Wasabi-Horseradish Dressing

 energizing | MAKES 2 TO 4 SERVINGS

Especially good in the late winter and early spring, when watercress appears in the cold streams and creeks and on the hillsides, this is a great revitalizing tonic salad with a fiery dressing that gets the blood moving after a sluggish winter. Eat this salad a couple of times a week throughout the spring—it's crunchy, spicy, and full of nutrients.

FOR THE SALAD

 1 handful of chopped fresh spinach

 2 handfuls of chopped fresh watercress, larger stems removed

 1 handful of fresh sugar snap peas

 2 to 3 red radishes, sliced

FOR THE DRESSING

 ¼ cup extra-virgin olive oil

 ½ cup yogurt

 ¼ teaspoon wasabi powder

 1 tablespoon prepared horseradish (from a jar), or to taste

 2 tablespoons lemon juice

To make the salad, tear the spinach into bite-size shreds and place in a large salad bowl with the watercress, peas, and radishes.

To make the dressing, whisk together all the dressing ingredients in a small bowl or jar and adjust quantities to taste. Pour the dressing over the salad and toss. Serve immediately.

WATERCRESS AND NASTURTIUM

Nasturtium officinale and *Tropaeolum majus*

A classic spring herb, watercress is that spicy, peppery green found along creeks and streams when winter gives way to spring. Its mustard oil content provides its characteristic sharp taste (even stronger than arugula), and it is rich in minerals, making it a traditional "spring tonic" in Appalachia and other North American regions. It combines well with lettuces, chickweed, and violets. Eat it raw or lightly steamed with vinegar.

Garden nasturtium, that lovely spicy herb with yellow, orange, or red flowers, is not related to watercress but was given the common name nasturtium in homage to the genus watercress belongs to. High in vitamin C, the many cultivated varieties of nasturtium can be eaten raw, mixed into salads, sautéed, pickled, and infused into vinegars—especially warming vinegars to be used during a cold or the flu.

HORSERADISH

Armoracia rusticana

Long used in traditional folk medicine and as a food source, horseradish is virtually forgotten today as a valid and reliable medicine. It is one of those medicines that quickly displays its actions: while the root is being grated, when it is eaten, or when the tinctured medicine is ingested, it quickly opens sinus passageways to relieve congestion. It is being studied for antibacterial properties. For sore muscles, the fresh raw root can be grated and made into a poultice similar to a poultice of fresh or ground mustard seeds. Include horseradish in vinegars and syrups, and experiment with it in pestos.

Crunchy Mint and Cucumber Salad

 digestive support | MAKES 2 TO 3 SERVINGS

Purslane delights in the summer with its slightly sweet, crunchy leaves and stems. I love snacking on it in the garden. Anise hyssop is another garden snack—I'll chew a pleasantly minty leaf as I work, and it always seems to wake me up. This recipe combine these flavors with mint and fresh, light cucumber for a crunchy, revitalizing salad. Picked in midmorning, before they wilt in the sun, these herbs will stay crunchy stored in the refrigerator (without the dressing) until lunchtime.

FOR THE SALAD

  1 handful of lettuce or spinach

  6 to 8 purslane leaves

  6 to 8 hyssop leaves, chopped

  1 small cucumber, seeded and chopped

  6 to 8 mint leaves, for garnish

FOR THE DRESSING

  ¼ cup olive or sunflower oil

  ½ cup white wine vinegar or lemon juice

  ½ cup yogurt

  1 tablespoon chopped fresh dill

  1 small cucumber, seeded and quartered

  Salt and ground black pepper, to taste

To make the salad, tear the lettuce into bite-size shreds and place in a large salad bowl with the whole purslane leaves, the hyssop, and the cucumber.

   To make the dressing, blend the olive oil, white wine vinegar, yogurt, dill, and cucumber in a blender until the cucumber is almost incorporated but there are still a few chunks. Add salt and pepper to taste. Pour the dressing over the salad and toss. Garnish with the mint leaves and serve immediately.

Lemony Vitality Salad and Dressing

 energizing | MAKES TWO 1-CUP SERVINGS

Tart, tangy, and lemony, this salad is a refreshing green treat.

FOR THE SALAD

  2 handfuls of your favorite lettuce

  1 handful of fat, crunchy purslane leaves

  1 handful of wood sorrel tops

  Toppings of your choice, such as chopped carrots and tomatoes

FOR THE DRESSING

  ⅓ cup olive or sunflower oil

HYSSOP

Hyssopus officinalis

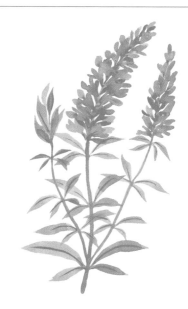

This lovely herb grows taller than many people and branches out from the base to create a picturesque and fragrant airy shrub. The edible leaves impart a bright, minty flavor, and it's a favorite of mine for snacking on in the garden. Medicinally, hyssop has long been used in the treatment of respiratory congestion, chronic catarrh, coughing, bronchitis, asthma, and colds. It is a mild expectorant and mild diaphoretic useful for children with colds, fevers, and influenza. Hyssop is also considered a nervine tonic, and interest in this herb is growing for its effects on stress, anxiety, and nervous tension. It works well as a tea or infusion and in syrups, and is a delight in honeys. Try chopping a tiny bit into tabbouleh for a refreshing mint flavor.

PURSLANE

Portulaca oleracea

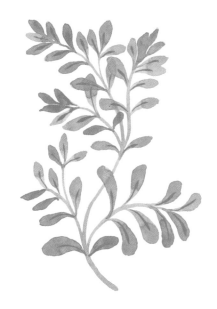

A weed in many parts of the world, purslane is a small succulent herb that spreads from one central point and sends out prostrate branches laden with fat, crunchy leaves. These leaves and stems are delicious and juicy, and they are extremely rich in omega-3 fatty acids. Purslane grows wild all over my garden, and I let some of the larger ones grow freely all summer; they get quite large (several feet in diameter), but the leaves must be harvested by midsummer or they begin to shrivel. Because of its nutrients and omega-3 content, purslane can be enjoyed for mental clarity and nervous system support, as well as for clear skin and general health. Eat it raw in salads or by itself, or steam it like spinach. Include a few chopped leaves in stews and soups.

3 tablespoons freshly squeezed lemon juice

2 teaspoons dried chopped lemongrass

1 teaspoon crumbled dried lemon balm

1 teaspoon crumbled dried lemon verbena

Dash each of salt and ground black pepper

To make the salad, tear the lettuce into bite-size shreds and place in a large salad bowl with the purslane leaves, wood sorrel, and toppings of your choice.

To make the dressing, put all the dressing ingredients into a small jar with a lid, cap, and shake to combine. Pour the dressing over the salad and toss. Serve immediately.

Child's Flower Fairy Salad

 nourishing | MAKES ABOUT 4 SERVINGS

For those special tea parties under the fairy bower, let the children harvest these colorful flowers and arrange a salad that no Fairy Queen could refuse. Place them in a large wooden salad bowl and offer a dish of salt and a bottle of dressing so each child can serve the next child at the table.

FOR THE SALAD

1 large handful of arugula, lettuce, or spinach

2 large handfuls of fresh mixed herbs—choose from the following:

Violet flowers and violet leaves (tiny new ones)

Borage flowers and leaves

Bee balm petals

Calendula petals

Nasturtium flowers

Fennel leaves

Chickweed tips (the stems get stringy)

FOR THE DRESSING

½ cup extra-virgin olive oil

¾ cup balsamic vinegar

1 tablespoon yogurt or sour cream

1 teaspoon honey

Salt and ground black pepper, to taste

To make the salad, tear the arugula into bite-size shreds and place them in a large wooden salad bowl with a combination of as many herbs as you wish.

To make the dressing, blend the olive oil, balsamic vinegar, yogurt, and honey in a blender or whisk in a bowl until smooth and lightly creamy. Add salt and pepper to taste. Serve the dressing on the side, or pour over the salad and toss. Enjoy immediately.

Borage, Fennel, and Raisin Salad
with Tangy Dressing

 nourishing | MAKES FOUR 1-CUP SERVINGS

This salad is a delight for the eyes: gather gorgeous, star-shaped blue borage flowers and pair them with bronze fennel and golden raisins. The turmeric in the dressing is optional, but it creates a striking yellow vinaigrette.

4 large handfuls of fresh mixed greens—choose from the following:

Borage leaves	Purslane leaves
Fennel leaves	Basil leaves
Lettuce	Spinach
Kale	Tender chard
Lamb's-quarter leaves	

1 cup fresh mixed flowers—choose from the following:

Red clover	Kale flowers
Collard flowers	Borage flowers

½ cup golden raisins

FOR THE DRESSING

⅓ cup extra-virgin olive oil

¼ cup fruity balsamic vinegar or lemon juice

½ teaspoon ground turmeric (for color), optional

1 teaspoon honey

To make the salad, combine the mixed greens in a large salad bowl. Tear any large pieces into bite-size shreds. Sprinkle the mixed flowers on top.

To make the dressing, whisk together all the dressing ingredients in a small bowl or jar. Drizzle over the salad and toss.

12

BROTHS AND SOUPS

Soup may well be the most ancient type of meal prepared by people. It's simple—so simple, in fact, that the tale of Stone Soup bears witness to its basic poverty. The tradition of *la cucina povera* of Italy attests to the adoration people have for soup, its simplicity of form and depth of flavor. But simple doesn't mean lacking—far from it. Soup (including broth, chowder, stew, stock, consommé, and bisque) can be wildly creative and fundamentally cultural. Every culture and country has its favorite method that it has refined over centuries.

We eat soup partly because it is simple, and partly because it makes us feel good. Soup is healing, fortifying, revitalizing. Soup is *restorative*—and in fact behind this very word is the French story of soup's role in the destiny of the modern restaurant:

> In 1765 a man by the name of Boulanger, also known as
> "Champ d'Oiseaux" or "Chantoiseau," opened a shop near the
> Louvre.... There he sold what he called *restaurants* or *bouil-*
> *lons restaurants*—that is, meat-based consommés intended
> to "restore" a person's strength. Ever since the late Middle
> Ages the word *restaurant* had been used to describe any of a

variety of rich bouillons made with chicken, beef, roots of one sort or another, onions, herbs, and, according to some recipes, spices, crystallized sugar, toasted bread, barley, butter, and even exotic ingredients such as dried rose petals, Damascus grapes, and amber.[1]

For centuries, meat-based soups have been used to fortify and restore, and the addition of various herbs, spices, flowers, roots, and fruits has carried this ancient culinary tradition into the present, yielding remarkable variety, flavor, and cultural subtleties for both meat and meatless soups and broths.

Herbs can be stars in soups and broths; simply tie sprigs in bundles that can be removed after cooking, let them steep in thin muslin bags, or chop them fine and let them become part of the texture of the final product as well as the taste. Experiment with using leaves (bay, thyme, yarrow, catnip, nettle, lemongrass), flowers (calendula, red clover, fennel, chive), stalks (celery, anise, fennel, savory), roots and tubers (astragalus, elecampane, yellow dock, dandelion, ginger), and bulbs (garlic, onion, Jerusalem artichoke). You can achieve slightly sweet overtones, depth, richness, earthiness, or clarity depending on which herbs you highlight in your soup. Always start small and work your way up for flavor.

BROTHS AND STOCKS

Bone broths and herbal broths are healing. When you're feeling low, fortify yourself by sipping a hot broth and letting it sink into your bones. Bone broths yield valuable collagen protein, heme iron (which is found only in animal ingredients), and minerals. Herbal and vegetable broths provide vitamins and have a healing factor that has yet to be identified but has been appreciated for generations. Plants contain tannins, saponins, flavonoids, resins, oils, polyphenols, bitters, and many other compounds that are extracted into the water that becomes the broth. Together these create a whole approach to eating and healing that is tasty and fortifying.

Broths are generally the same thing as stocks and bouillon: they are clear, and all solids have been removed. Sip your broth fresh and hot, or store it in a Thermos to enjoy all day long.

---

1. Jean-Robert Pitte, "The Rise of the Restaurant," in Albert Sonnenfeld (ed.), *Food: A Culinary History from Antiquity to the Present* (New York: Columbia University Press, 1999).

FENNEL

Foeniculum vulgare

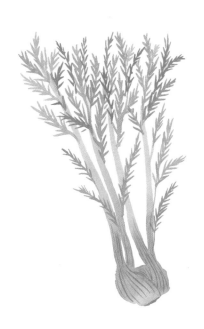

An ancient herb, fennel has been used for centuries in both the kitchen and the medicine cabinet. Nursing mothers have long used fennel in their mixtures to bring on breast-milk flow and increase production, and have given it to their babies to reduce spastic colon and colic. Adults and children like to nibble on fresh fennel leaves, indulge in candied dried fennel seeds, or use fresh or dried fennel leaves and seeds in tinctures to relieve acute indigestion, ulcer, food cravings, gas, bloating and distension, and constipation. In the broth recipes in this book, fennel fronds are used, and the seeds are best used in honeys and teas and ground into salt blends.

Clear Fennel Broth

 immune support | YIELDS 1 QUART

This lovely broth celebrates the flavor of fennel, with its hint of anise, and it pairs well with light spring and summer meals that feature tomatoes, asparagus, and baguettes. It can also be part of a more substantial meal: add depth of flavor to its light texture by stewing bones, meats, potatoes, and seaweeds. Strain it well after cooking to make a healing broth to sip when you're feeling under the weather.

1 tablespoon extra-virgin olive oil

½ yellow onion, coarsely chopped

5 garlic cloves, peeled and coarsely chopped

¼ cup fennel seeds

2 to 3 fresh fennel leaves, optional

2 to 3 fresh chive flower heads, or 1 teaspoon dried chopped chives

2 bay leaves

4 cups water

Salt and ground black pepper, to taste

Heat the olive oil in a medium saucepan over medium heat. Add the onion and garlic and cook, stirring continuously, until the onion is translucent, 3 to 4 minutes. Don't allow the garlic to burn! Add the fennel seeds, fennel leaves (if using), chives, and bay leaves and cook, stirring, for 1 minute.

Pour in the water and increase the heat until it comes to a slow simmer. Simmer, stirring occasionally, for 15 minutes. Add salt and pepper to taste, then either strain into serving bowls to sip hot or use as a base for other soups.

Thai Lemongrass Broth

 immune support | YIELDS ABOUT 2 QUARTS

This light, tangy broth is an immune-supportive powerhouse, wonderful to sip when there's a cough or flu in the family. Inspired by the traditional Thai *tom yung kung* soup, which is a favorite in our family, this soup brings in dried herbs that go the distance. Astragalus is traditionally used for long-term immune support, and the optional angelica is a respiratory aid with a pleasant anise-like flavor. This is served as a broth, so all solids will be removed before serving. Go heavy on the herbs in this broth to get the full flavor, adding lemon or lime juice right before serving.

2 tablespoons extra-virgin olive oil

10 to 15 button or crimini mushrooms, chopped

5 garlic cloves, minced

1-inch piece of fresh gingerroot, minced

1-inch piece of fresh angelica root, chopped, or 1 teaspoon dried, optional

Two 2-inch pieces of dried astragalus root, chopped

1 tablespoon dried chopped lemongrass, or 1 to 2 teaspoons frozen lemongrass concentrate

2 quarts water

Handful of fresh parsley leaves, or 2 teaspoons crumbled dried parsley

Salt and ground black pepper, to taste

2 teaspoons lemon or lime juice per serving

Heat the olive oil in a large saucepan over medium heat and cook the mushrooms, garlic, ginger, angelica (if using), astragalus, and lemongrass, stirring frequently, for about 5 minutes. Add the water, increase the heat, and bring to a boil. Reduce the heat to low and simmer until the roots have softened, 15 to 20 minutes. Add the parsley at the very end. Add salt and pepper to taste, then strain into serving bowls. Add the lemon juice and serve hot.

Spicy Ginger Broth

 immune support | YIELDS 1 PINT

This is a medicinal broth to be prepared for someone feeling under the weather. Making only 2 cups, this recipe will give you enough broth for the patient to sip from a Thermos throughout the day but not enough for a whole meal. However, the broth can become part of a larger recipe such as an Indian or Thai soup.

3 cups water

3-inch piece of fresh gingerroot, chopped

4 to 6 garlic cloves, peeled and cut in half

1 teaspoon whole peppercorns

1 teaspoon fennel seeds

¼ teaspoon cayenne pepper, or to taste

Juice of ½ lemon

Zest of ½ lemon

Salt, to taste

Combine the water, ginger, garlic, peppercorns, fennel seeds, cayenne, lemon juice, and lemon zest in a medium saucepan over high heat. Bring to a boil, then reduce the heat to low and simmer, stirring occasionally, until the liquid has reduced to about 2 cups and the broth is fragrant, 20 to 30 minutes. Strain into a Thermos.

Wild Greens Miso Paste by Kate Gilday

 nourishing | YIELDS ABOUT 2 CUPS

Most miso is a fermented soy paste that is diluted and added to soup. This special, uncooked paste by the herbalist Kate Gilday uses just a little soy miso while it highlights a variety of wild, flavorful herbs that add depth and nuance to your favorite broths. Kate suggests adding this miso paste to flavor soups and stews or to thicken tomato sauce and even suggests spreading it over chicken as a marinade before grilling. It can be made through the seasons with different edible wild greens you can find in and out of the garden. Kate notes that it freezes well, but it should be used within 6 months or so for the best flavor and nutrition. "Use an ice cube tray to freeze small amounts or small yogurt containers for larger amounts," she says.

Kate recommends using any of the following greens and preparing them ahead of time, and encourages you to use your imagination as you blend different tastes and flavors. In the spring, try violet leaf, early plantain leaves, dandelion leaves, nettle leaves, wild mustard leaves and/or flower buds, a small amount of daisy leaves (before the plant flowers), garlic mustard leaves (garlic scapes are nice later in the summer), wild onion, and chives. In the summer, use lamb's-quarters, nettles, purslane, galinsoga, pigweed, garlic, and chives.

½ cup extra-virgin olive oil

¼ cup miso (white for a milder flavor, aduki bean for a more pronounced flavor)

1 tablespoon minced fresh "savory" herbs, such as seaweed, garlic, rosemary, basil, and/or thyme, optional

4 cups roughly chopped fresh herbs and leaves of your choice (see suggestions above)

Blend the olive oil, miso, and savory herbs, if desired, in a blender or food processor. With the blender running, add the other herbs and leaves a little at a time until you reach a paste-like consistency. To use in soup or broth, whisk in 1 to 2 teaspoons of paste per cup of soup when soup is ready to serve. Store in an airtight glass container in the refrigerator for up to 4 weeks or in the freezer for up to 6 months.

Medicinal Mushroom Stock

by Robin Rose Bennett

 immune support | YIELDS ABOUT 1 QUART

The herbalist Robin Rose Bennett says, "Some medicinal mushrooms, such as reishi, turkey tails, and chaga, are too hard and woody to eat, so these are removed after cooking. They can be mixed with other dried, edible mushrooms and prepared in a pot to make a mushroom stock." Robin notes that all mushrooms intended to be eaten, dried or fresh, should be cooked: "This breaks down the chitins and lignins that make up a mushroom's cell wall. (In contrast to mushrooms, plants' cell walls are made up of digestible cellulose.)" The key to making this stock successful, she says, is very long steeping on very low heat: "I steep my mushroom or mushroom-and-vegetable stock for about 24 hours, either on the lowest possible heat on the gas stove, or on a trivet on top of the woodstove." It is then strained and squeezed out, and can be eaten on its own or used to cook other dishes that normally require cooking water. Robin likes to use this stock in her Bone Soup (page 202).

1 cup sliced reishi mushrooms

¾ cup sliced chaga

¾ cup sliced turkey tail mushrooms

4 cups water

In a small, heavy-bottomed pot set over low heat, sear the mushrooms, stirring occasionally. Add the water and gently heat for 24 to 48 hours, according to taste. Strain through cheesecloth, then gather up the cloth around the mushrooms and squeeze to extract as much broth as possible. Compost the mushrooms. Use immediately or store in an airtight container in the freezer.

Deep Healing Chicken Herb Broth

 immune support | YIELDS 3 TO 4 QUARTS

There is something to the traditional chicken soup remedy! In our house, when someone is feeling sick, we get a chicken (one we've raised or one we've purchased) and make a big pot of chicken soup, usually with vegetables and rice. If someone really can't bear to eat but has hunger pangs, the broth alone is easier to digest, tastes delicious, and is still infused with strong healing herbs that support the immune system. This broth can be used as the basis of soup or sipped on its own; then use the cooked chicken meat to make a healthy meal.

1 small whole chicken (3 to 5 pounds)

3 to 4 quarts water

1 tablespoon *each* crushed dried oregano, thyme, rosemary, and sage (or a *bouquet garni* of sprigs of these fresh herbs tied in a bundle)

3 bay leaves

1 teaspoon fennel seeds

Salt and ground black pepper, to taste

Rinse the chicken and remove any giblets or feathers. Place the chicken in a medium pot and fill with 3 to 4 quarts water, enough to cover it by an inch or so. Add the dried herbs or tuck the *bouquet garni* in beside the chicken. Add the bay leaves and fennel seeds. Turn the heat to high and place a lid loosely over the pot. When the mixture is close to boiling, reduce the heat to low and simmer until the chicken is cooked through and the meat pulls easily off the bones, 30 to 40 minutes.

At this point, most of the herbs will be floating, and you'll notice a lot of oily bubbles on the surface. Together with the herb-infused water, this fat is what makes the broth so special. Carefully lift the chicken from the pot, place on a plate, and set aside for another use. (Allow it to cool, then remove the meat from the bones and use in soup or another meal.) Using a ladle, pour the broth through a strainer into 1-quart glass canning jars. (You will probably fill three to four 1-quart jars.) Be sure to pour some of the broth into a serving bowl to enjoy while it's fresh and hot. Store the rest in the refrigerator for up to 2 weeks. Alternatively, ladle into freezer-safe containers and freeze for up to 6 months.

Venison Broth with Oregano and Thyme

 immune support | YIELDS 1 PINT

My husband and son are part of a community that hunts the many deer here on Martha's Vineyard Island. When they bring home a deer, we process it in our kitchen, preparing all the many cuts of meat and using the bones and other parts to make broth. We freeze the meat and can the broth using a pressure canner and glass canning jars. Rocco and I use the venison

OREGANO AND THYME

Origanum vulgare and *Thymus vulgaris*

Common oregano and thyme have been used since ancient times for healing wounds and disinfecting the lungs. Each can be burned to purify the air and smoked as part of a smoking mixture, and both have been used as meat preservatives. Because oregano is very strong and can cause stomach upset in large doses, it is best to use it medicinally only for specific conditions; for general use, it can be used topically or eaten as a spice. Thyme is often enjoyed as a tea. Although neither herb is a tonic in the true sense, each can be used for specific instances where immune support is needed, as a chewed herb, a fresh herb in cooking, in broths and soups, and infused into honey.

broth all winter for soups, stews, and gravies. Its strong flavor combines well with the immune-supporting herbs thyme and oregano to create a powerful healing broth, which can be enjoyed in meals or as a medicinal broth to sip during cold and flu season. If you don't have venison broth, use chicken, turkey, or beef broth.

> 3 cups venison broth or other broth
> ½ cup fresh oregano leaves, or 2 tablespoons crushed dried
> ½ cup fresh thyme leaves, or 2 tablespoons crushed dried
> 1 teaspoon whole peppercorns
> 1 teaspoon dried rosemary leaves
> Salt, to taste

Combine the venison broth, oregano, thyme, peppercorns, and rosemary in a medium saucepan over high heat. Bring to a low boil, then reduce the heat to low and simmer until the liquid has reduced to about 2 cups and the broth is fragrant, 20 to 30 minutes. Stir occasionally, and skim off any fat that rises to the top. (I like to give this to our dog as a treat.) Strain into a Thermos.

SOUP

Thick and chunky, or watery and spicy, soups come in all forms. The soups included here are dense with nutrition, and they use ingredients that we should all try to include in our diets more often—wild and rich and green, fresh from the fields and garden and ocean. If you can't find a particular green, feel free to substitute spinach, but by all means try to use the nettles and seaweeds called for here—your body will thank you.

These soups include berries and leaves as well as mushrooms, fish, seaweeds, and herbs. They are hearty and healing and can be made for a special friend on a special occasion, or they can become part of your family's repertoire to nourish you weekly through a long winter.

Nettle Soup by Corinna Wood

 iron-rich | YIELDS 2 QUARTS

"When hungry faces surround my table," says the herbalist Corinna Wood, "I like to prepare a hearty meal that nourishes body and soul. This rich, buttery nettle soup hits the spot. Serve it up with some brown rice or bread and butter, and it will provide plenty of energy for an afternoon among the herbs, or an evening of great conversation with friends and family."

- 2 tablespoons extra-virgin olive oil
- 1 medium onion, chopped
- 2 garlic cloves, minced
- 1 cup diced carrots
- 1 cup diced potatoes
- 6 cups water or vegetable or chicken broth
- 3 cups fresh nettle tops
- Sweet white miso, to taste

Heat the olive oil in a medium pot over medium heat. Add the onion and garlic and cook, stirring often, until the onion is translucent, about 5 minutes. Stir in the carrots and potatoes and cook for about 3 minutes, then cover with the water or broth. Add the nettle tops and bring to a boil. (If your nettle tops are small, you can put them in whole. If they're larger than would fit on your spoon, put on gloves and chop them coarsely before adding to the soup.) When boiling, reduce the heat to low and simmer until carrots and potatoes are tender, 35 to 45 minutes.

Take about 2 tablespoons hot broth (plus some cold water) out of the pot and combine it in a small bowl with enough cold water to bring it to a tepid temperature. Whisk in several spoonfuls of miso and set aside. Ladle the cooked soup into bowls and serve. Add the diluted miso to the bowls of soup at the table so the miso's live beneficial microorganisms don't get killed by the boiling temperature of the soup.

Scandinavian Nettle Soup with Fish

by Hank Shaw

 nourishing | YIELDS ABOUT 2 QUARTS

The *Hunt, Gather, Cook* author Hank Shaw describes this as a mash-up between a traditional Swedish *nässelsoppa* nettle soup and a smooth French-style fish bisque, and he says you can't get any greener than this soup. The flavors are warm, smooth, and alive—bright, clean, and briny. He says that any lean white fish works, but you don't want to use an oily fish here. If you don't have access to nettles, use a fifty-fifty mix of parsley and spinach for a similar effect. The greens must be blanched before you use them in this soup. You can use frozen, cooked spinach, but you'll need to blanch the parsley for 1 minute in salty, boiling water and then shock it in an ice bath. Nettles need to blanch for anywhere from 30 to 90 seconds in the boiling water.

Don't be tempted to use fish broth for this soup, says Hank. "You want the fishy flavor to be subtle. I use homemade pheasant broth for my soup, but I would also recommend chicken or vegetable broth. Finally, you don't have to strain the soup after pureeing it. I do, because I like refined soups. But it will be fine to eat right out of the blender."

- 3 tablespoons unsalted butter
- 1 cup chopped white onion
- 1 garlic clove, minced
- 4 cups chicken or vegetable stock
- 1 teaspoon dried thyme leaves
- ½ teaspoon freshly grated nutmeg, plus more to taste
- Pinch of salt, plus more to taste
- 1 pound lean white fish (such as cod, bass, tilapia, shark, or walleye), roughly chopped
- 1 pound nettles, blanched and chopped (or substitute parsley and spinach together)
- Sour cream and ground black pepper, for garnish

Heat the butter in a large saucepan over medium heat. Add the onion and cook, stirring often, until they are soft and translucent. Add the garlic and cook 1 minute more. Pour in the stock and add the thyme, nutmeg, salt, fish, and blanched nettles. Bring to a gentle boil, then reduce the heat to low and simmer until the nettles are very tender, 15 to 20 minutes. Taste the soup and add more salt and/or nutmeg if it needs it. You want to be able to taste the nutmeg in the final dish.

Puree the soup in a blender. You might need to do this in batches. Then, if you want to get fancy, push the puree through a fine-mesh sieve over another pot or a bowl. Return the pureed or pureed and strained soup to the saucepan and place over low heat until just warmed through. Serve in bowls with a dollop of sour cream and sprinkled with black pepper.

Bone Soup by Robin Rose Bennett

 immune support | YIELD VARIES

The herbalist Robin Rose Bennett says she enjoys this bone soup recipe consistently and recommends it for both preventive and curative medicine. "I consider bone soup to be a life-sustaining, immune-strengthening tonic, and one of the best food medicines available to us," she says. "Making bone broths, consommés, and soups releases nutrients (especially iron) from the bones, the marrow, and any meat left on the bone. It replenishes us, aiding our overburdened endocrine systems and helping us recover when we feel depleted and exhausted." Robin suggests using medicinal mushrooms or the Medicinal Mushroom Stock (page 197) in this bone soup for a true powerhouse of a restorative meal.

"Any version of this soup will warm and heal you deep inside your bone marrow," says Robin. "Use it as a strengthening tonic throughout the fall and winter, or eat one or two bowls daily when healing from serious conditions."

1 large bone with meat on it, such as a cow shin bone

4 cups of saved bones from any animal, preferably free-range or pasture-raised and organically fed (see note)

¼ cup mushroom vinegar, apple cider, or infused herbal vinegar

1½ cups dried sliced astragalus root

1 cup seaweed of choice, plus more if desired

OPTIONAL ADDITIONS

2 to 4 cups chopped vegetables (such as carrots, mushrooms, celery, onions, leeks, and/or leafy greens), sautéed

Herbs and spices, such as marjoram, garlic, ginger, turmeric, cinnamon, and/or salt, to taste

1 cup Medicinal Mushroom Stock (page 197), plus more if desired

1 cup dried mushrooms, such as reishi, chaga, or turkey tail

½ cup crumbled dried nettle leaves

If using the optional shin bone, preheat the oven to 350°F. Put the bone in a large soup pot and roast it for 1 to 1½ hours, until the meat is tender and falls off the bone. If the bone has been frozen, put it in a roasting pan and place in the oven to thaw and roast while you prepare the rest of the soup. (You can add it to the soup after it's roasted, so you can start your soup right away, without waiting for it to thaw.)

Add the saved bones to the soup pot (handling the pot carefully if it's been in a hot oven) and add enough cold water, or a combination of cold water and mushroom or vegetable stock, to cover by 1 inch. Next, add the mushroom vinegar to help draw out the minerals in the bones. Put the pot over high heat and bring to a boil, then reduce the heat to low and simmer for 2 to 3 hours.

Add the astragalus and seaweed—these are the final essential ingredients; the rest are optional. To stop here, simmer the soup over low heat on your stovetop or on a trivet on a woodstove for another 12 to 48 hours, according to taste. The long, slow steeping brings out the gelatin and protein from the bones.

If you'd like to include chopped vegetables, add them in the last 8 to 12 hours of cooking. This is also the time to add a few dashes of warming winter spices such as ginger, turmeric, and cinnamon. Robin loves to add marjoram, finding that its sweetness helps balance the other flavors.

When you've waited as long as you can and you feel the soup is done, strain it, making sure the marrow has come out of the bones. Discard any cooked vegetables with the bones and herbs, or pick them out and return them to the soup. Alternatively, puree the vegetables in a blender with some of the broth and then return the mixture to the pot. Adjust the seasonings to your taste. Refrigerate some for immediate use, and freeze the rest in labeled freezer containers. This broth can be enjoyed as is or used as the cooking liquid in rice and other dishes.

NOTE: I accumulate a combination of various types of bones in one large, sealable plastic bag or jar in my freezer until I have enough to make soup. I don't clean them of scraps or gristle, as the soup will get strained.

ASTRAGALUS

Astragalus membranaceus

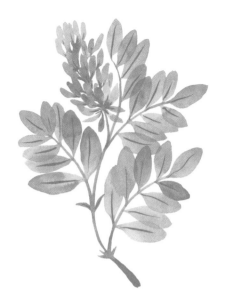

Used for thousands of years throughout Asia as both a food and a medicine, astragalus is one of the safest immune-supporting herbs we know, as well as one of the most potent. Rich in glycosides and polysaccharides, astragalus is commonly used to stimulate and support the immune system, and for this its root has shown strong activity in-vitro, in laboratory settings, in folklore, and in clinical settings. The herbal researcher Stephen Harrod Buhner reports that it protects the heart from the Coxsackie B2 virus and prevents cancer metastasis. Other researchers report that it supports the body's efforts to remove unwanted foreign materials, enhances stem-cell production, and protects the liver against certain toxins. Astragalus is generally used to support the pituitary gland and restore depleted red-blood-cell formation in bone marrow, and its white fibrous roots are often included in remedies to support immunity, combat Lyme disease, and protect against viral infection. Its bland and unassuming flavor means it can be used abundantly in teas, decoctions, stews, soups, broths, herb powder blends, honeys, and syrups.

13

MAIN DISHES

Greens and herbs feature brightly in these main dishes. Using nettles, lamb's-quarters, and parsley is a great way to bring the fresh vibrant qualities of wild and garden herbs into the kitchen. Nettles are famously high in vitamins and minerals, and after they are cooked their juices become a pot-liquor that can be drunk as a fortifying tea (see Nettle sidebar, page 206).

Nettles and greens lend themselves to delicious pasta dinners and to meals with a variety of grains, such as millet, couscous, barley, and rice. Make the following sautés to taste, and experiment with serving them on different grains topped with a simple miso gravy (such as Wild Greens Miso Paste, page 196) or a sprinkling of olive oil (such as Mineral-Rich Seaweed Oil for Cooking, page 37, or A-to-Z Warming Oil, page 39) and either lemon juice or ume plum vinegar.

NETTLE
Urtica dioica

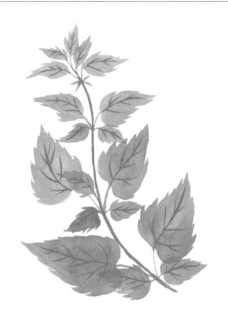

One of the most nourishing and versatile herbs I know, stinging nettle has become one of Western herbalism's most beloved herbs. The mineral-rich leaves are extremely high in calcium, magnesium, iron, trace minerals, protein, and chlorophyll, making this herb ideal for use during pregnancy, breast-feeding, and menopause, and in cases of anemia. It grows in cool, rich woodlands and is easy to harvest with gloves; its stinging hairs contain formic acid and histamine, which are injected into people or animals when they brush against it (hence the name *nettle,* or needle), resulting in a temporary, stinging rash.

Try delicious nettle leaves as an infusion or infused in vinegar, olive oil, or honey. Enjoy pureed nettles alone, mixed into cream cheese, or infused into a rich pudding.

Nettle and Onion Skillet with Rice

 iron-rich | MAKES 3 TO 4 SERVINGS

My husband taught me the value of the size of the chop: leaving vegetables big makes a big difference in the flavor of a sauté. My tendency is to mince vegetables, and as a result they get mushy. But he cuts them into big chunks, and this translates into a beautiful sauté dish with lots of crunch and flavor. Cut your onion in slices that seem larger than you think they should be; they'll soften and shrink just a bit and will taste delicious. This dish is a delightful way to enjoy the deep, earthy flavor of wild greens.

Serve the sautéed vegetables on top of steaming-hot rice with a fresh salad, such as the Red Cabbage and Arame Salad (page 184) or the Summer Solstice Salad (page 180). Reserve any liquid that is left over in the skillet to drizzle on top before serving.

FOR THE RICE

1½ cups long-grain rice (such as wild rice or basmati)

3 cups water, broth, or stock (such as Medicinal Mushroom Stock, page 197)

FOR THE SAUTÉ

2 tablespoons extra-virgin olive oil

½ large onion (preferably Vidalia or a flavorful yellow onion), cut into half-moon chunks

4 to 6 large handfuls of fresh, young nettle leaves

1 cup other quick-cooking vegetables (such as cherry tomatoes, asparagus tips, or shelled peas), optional

Salt and ground black pepper, to taste

To make the rice, put the rice into a small saucepan over medium heat and cook, stirring frequently, until the rice smells fragrant. Add the water and stir once more, then cover tightly with a lid. Bring to a boil, then reduce the heat to low and cook until all the liquid has absorbed, about 20 minutes. Remove the pan from the heat and set aside.

To make the sauté while the rice is cooking, heat a medium cast iron skillet over medium-high heat. Pour the olive oil into the skillet, add the onion, and sauté, stirring occasionally, until the edges of the onions are translucent and soft. Meanwhile, using gloved hands, mound the nettle leaves on a cutting board and give them two or three coarse chops. Add the nettles to the pan along with any other quick-cooking vegetables, if desired, and sauté until the nettle leaves are bright green and tender. Season with salt and pepper.

Transfer the cooked rice onto a serving platter and ladle the sautéed vegetables on top, then drizzle any leftover liquid from the skillet on top. Serve hot.

Wild Green Sauté with Polenta and Poached Egg

 iron-rich | MAKES 3 SERVINGS

When you eat steamed greens, it feels like you are building your bones. It feels substantial, like you've climbed a mountain or finished a big project. A big, hot bowl of lightly steamed greens drizzled with vinegar and sprinkled with flaky salt and freshly ground pepper—it is the motivation and it is the reward. Enjoy these greens for their iron, fiber, vitamins A, B6, C, and K, folate, calcium, copper, and manganese. But especially enjoy them for their spectacular flavor.

The polenta can be made using millet or corn grits, and the egg can be poached or hard-boiled. Together, these make a satisfying and very nutritious main dish. Alternatively, use these sautéed greens as a side dish to a main meal, as a snack, or even as a fortifying breakfast when you don't want something sweet.

FOR THE POLENTA

- 1 cup millet or corn grits
- 3 cups water, broth, or stock
- ¼ teaspoon salt

FOR THE SAUTÉ

- 6 cups roughly chopped fresh greens, such as young nettle leaves, spinach, kale, collard greens, turnip greens, Swiss chard, and/or lamb's-quarters
- ½ cup water
- 1 tablespoon extra-virgin olive oil
- 2 tablespoons balsamic or apple cider vinegar
- Salt and ground black pepper, to taste

3 poached or hard-boiled eggs

If using millet, grind it in a blender to the consistency of grits. To make the polenta, pour the millet or corn grits into a medium saucepan over medium heat and cook, stirring frequently, until thick and creamy. Add the water and salt, stir once more, then cover tightly with a lid. Bring to a boil, then reduce the heat to low and cook until all the liquid has absorbed, about 20 minutes. Divide the polenta among 3 plates.

Meanwhile, to make the sauté, heat a wide skillet or wok over medium-high heat. Place the greens in the skillet in one massive heap, pour the water over them, and quickly cover with a lid. Steam for 1 minute, then carefully remove the lid and stir, making sure the leaves don't stick on the pan. Cook, stirring and fluffing continuously, until the greens are bright and have just started to wilt, 1 to 2 minutes.

Spoon the greens on top of the polenta. Drizzle the olive oil and balsamic vinegar over the top and season with salt and pepper. Top each plate with an egg, drizzle any leftover liquid from the skillet on top, and serve hot.

Tabbouleh with Parsley and Sautéed Tilapia

by Rosalee de la Forêt

 iron-rich | MAKES 6 SERVINGS

The herbalist and educator Rosalee de la Forêt shares her recipe for a simple summer tabbouleh that is chock-full of fresh veggies and herbs, especially parsley. "This dish is perfect for summer barbecues and potlucks," she says. "Tabbouleh recipes originally come from the eastern Mediterranean. There are thousands of versions out there. To make this my own recipe I added a generous amount of fresh fennel and switched out the glutinous bulgur or couscous for quinoa." Served with sautéed tilapia or other white fish, it makes for a delicious meal.

- 1 cup quinoa
- 2 cups water or vegetable broth
- 2 cups chopped fresh parsley leaves
- 2 cups chopped fennel bulb
- 6 green onions, chopped
- 1 cup sliced cherry tomatoes
- 1 cup diced cucumber
- ¼ cup chopped fresh mint leaves
- ½ cup freshly squeezed lemon juice (from about 3 lemons)
- Zest of 3 lemons
- ½ cup extra-virgin olive oil
- Salt and ground black pepper, to taste
- 1 tablespoon oil for searing the fish (choose from olive, grapeseed, safflower, and canola)
- ½ pound tilapia filets (or a similar white fish, such as cod or sea bass), cut into strips and patted dry
- Juice of 1 lemon or lime
- Paprika, for garnish

Rinse the quinoa well in a fine-mesh sieve. Combine the quinoa and water in a medium saucepan over high heat. Bring to a boil, then reduce the heat to low, cover, and simmer until the water has been absorbed and the quinoa is light and fluffy, 18 to 20 minutes. Allow to cool.

Once the quinoa has cooled, toss it in a large bowl along with the parsley, fennel, green onions, tomatoes, cucumber, and mint. Add the lemon juice, lemon zest, and olive oil. Stir well and season with salt and pepper. Set aside.

Heat a flat-bottomed skillet or griddle on medium to high heat. Add the oil, then lay the fish strips on the pan ¼ inch apart. Sear the strips for 2 or 3 minutes, then flip them with a spatula. Sear for another 3 minutes, then remove from the pan and place on top of the tabbouleh. Drizzle the fish and tabbouleh with the lemon juice and sprinkle with paprika. Serve hot, or chill the entire dish overnight and serve cold for a picnic lunch.

Ricotta Gnocchi and Carrot Broth
by Hank Shaw

 nourishing | MAKES 4 TO 6 SERVINGS

Hank Shaw, a cookbook author and the proprietor of the award-winning website *Hunter Angler Gardener Cook,* calls this delicious homemade pasta "the soul of simplicity," noting that he "typically uses cow parsnip for this recipe, but don't get all hung up on it." Cow parsnip leaves have the tang and bite of parsley or lovage, a flavor that pairs beautifully with the carrot broth. Hank says any wild green will do, including amaranth greens, borage, nettles, dandelions, lamb's-quarters, lovage, or even regular parsley. But he says you *should* get hung up on the timing of the gnocchi: make the dough right before you cook the dumplings, otherwise you will find you need much more flour to keep them intact, which will make your gnocchi heavier. The carrot broth can be made up to a day ahead.

"I serve this recipe either as part of a larger, longer meal or as a light summer dinner," says Hank. "You can fill yourself up on these gnocchi, but it's more fun to serve this soup with, say, a salad and some seared duck breast or a grilled steak. This is really not that hard a dish to make. Honest."

FOR THE BROTH
1 pound carrots, peeled and roughly chopped

5 cups water

Salt, to taste

FOR THE GNOCCHI
2 teaspoons salt

2 ounces young cow parsnip leaves or other young wild greens (about 15 to 20 small leaves), blanched and squeezed

1 pound whole milk ricotta cheese

½ cup finely grated pecorino or Parmesan cheese

½ teaspoon ground nutmeg

2 eggs, lightly beaten

Approximately 1½ cups all-purpose flour

To make the broth, pulse the carrots in a food processor until they are in little bits (but not pureed), or chop them finely. Put the minced carrots and the water in a medium saucepan over high heat. Bring to a boil, then reduce the heat to low and simmer for 20 minutes. Turn off the heat, cover the pan, and let the mixture steep for 1 hour.

Meanwhile, bring a large pot of water to a boil; this is what you'll cook the gnocchi in. Add enough salt to make it taste like the sea. Also prepare a medium bowl of ice water.

When the gnocchi water is boiling, add the cow parsnip leaves and cook for 2 minutes (most other wild greens will need only 1 minute). Remove the cow parsnip from the pot and submerge in the bowl of ice water to halt the cooking process. Take the chilled leaves out of the water, squeeze out any excess moisture, and mince well (but do not puree—unless you want green gnocchi, which is an option!). Keep the pot of water hot.

To make the gnocchi, put the cow parsnip, ricotta, pecorino, nutmeg, eggs, and the 2 teaspoons of salt in a large bowl and stir well to incorporate. Stir in enough of the flour that the dough comes together in a mass that can be kind of kneaded, but not really. It should be soft, pliable, and just a little sticky. The better you get at making gnocchi, the less flour you will need.

Flour your work surface well. Shape the gnocchi dough into a rough rectangle in the bowl and cut it into 4 equal pieces. Put a piece of dough on the work surface and gently roll it with your hands into a log a little less than 1 inch thick. You might need to cut the log into serviceable lengths to continue rolling.

Use a knife to cut the log into gnocchi dumplings about 1 inch long. They will look a little like pillows. Gently roll them in the flour to coat the cut edges. Set aside on a floured baking sheet and repeat the process until all the dough has been rolled and cut into dumplings.

Strain the steeped carrot broth through a fine-mesh sieve lined with cheesecloth or a paper towel into a separate, clean saucepan. Alternatively, strain into a medium bowl, clean out the saucepan, and return the strained broth to the pan.

To finish, heat the carrot broth over medium heat until it steams, but do not boil it. Add salt to taste. Carefully put all the gnocchi in the large pot of boiling water. Boil the gnocchi until they are floating, then cook for 1 minute more. Lift them out with a slotted spoon and transfer directly into individual bowls. Pour the carrot broth over the pasta and serve.

Lamb's-Quarter Cavatelli

 nourishing | MAKES 6 TO 8 SERVINGS

A key benefit of marrying into an Italian family is learning how to cook pasta; I've adapted this recipe from the family recipe belonging to my mother-in-law, Mary Bellebuono, and I roll the dough out on a large, antique board that was handmade by my husband's grandfather for his wife, Antoinette. My husband remembers visiting Antoinette when he was a child and watching her make a large batch of cavatelli by hand, using her fingers and a fork to roll each noodle, one by one, on the special wooden board. She probably used semolina and wheat flours; I've added some wild seed flour made from grinding dried lamb's-quarter seeds, which gives the pasta a bit of a darker color and a certain wild flavor from our garden.

Harvest the lamb's-quarter seeds by stripping the seeds off the branches into a paper bag, husks and all. Spread them on a newspaper to dry; once they've dried, grind them in a food processor or blender until they become a fine meal or flour. Collect about 3 cups of seeds to make 1 cup of lamb's-quarter flour. Freeze any unused lamb's-quarter flour and use it anytime you need extra flour or want a little wildness to come through in a recipe.

3 cups semolina flour

1 cup lamb's-quarter seed flour

½ cup white flour

1 egg

½ cup extra-virgin olive oil

1½ cups water

1 teaspoon salt, or to taste

Combine all the ingredients in a medium bowl and mix by hand until the dough is well combined and soft but holds together. If it's too loose, add more semolina; if it's too dry and thick, add more oil and water. Keep the ratio of semolina to combined other flours at about 2:1. Cover the dough with a damp cloth and allow to rest for 10 minutes.

Bring a large pot of salted water to a boil. With a rolling pin, roll the dough out on a floured work surface and slice it into 1-inch strips. Run the pasta strips through a pasta machine (I use a hand-crank cavatelli maker), or cut off 2-inch-long chunks and roll them into shape with a fork. Set them aside in a single layer on several floured baking sheets.

Salt the boiling water and add the cavatelli from about half of the baking sheet. Boil until all the noodles are floating in the pot, 5 to 8 minutes. Scoop the cavatelli out with a slotted spoon and place them in a saucepan. Drizzle with a little olive oil so they don't stick together. Repeat with the rest of the cavatelli, cooking it in batches.

The pasta will be a slight green color and a little darker than your normal pasta, thanks to the lamb's-quarter flour. These cavatelli are perfectly complemented by a crusty baguette and a crisp salad. Enjoy with tomato sauce, Wild Lamb's-Quarter Pesto (page 43), or Sage Butter (page 48) and topped with toasted walnuts or chestnuts.

LAMB'S-QUARTER

Chenopodium album

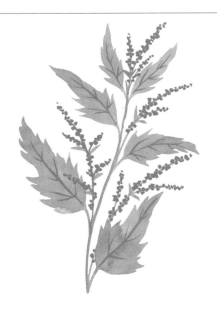

Related to quinoa, lamb's-quarters are the herbalist's crunchy, tasty, wild gift from the garden. These plants start as small, silvery-gray seedlings that grow to 7 or 8 feet high over the course of a season. They are spindly and wiry and gray, so they don't make a very attractive vegetable, but they are certainly nutritious. The leaves are used extensively in cuisines around the world, in curries, stews, breads, and sautés; the young shoots can be steamed and eaten like turnip greens, and the plentiful seeds can be easily stripped from the branches in the fall and dried. They make an excellent flour (from which you can make pastas and breads), and they give a satisfying crunch when baked with crackers or sprinkled on oatmeal. The seeds are high in protein, vitamin A, calcium, and other minerals, and they store well after being dried. Use the seeds abundantly; use the leaves in addition to other leafy vegetables but not alone in large quantities since, like spinach and wood sorrel, they are high in oxalic acid.

Nettle Ravioli by Jan Buhrman

 iron-rich | MAKES 6 TO 8 SERVINGS

Vineyard chef and caterer Jan Buhrman uses nettles wherever she can. Here, nettles and ricotta cheese form both the filling and the structure for delicious homemade raviolis.

FOR THE PASTA

    4 cups durum semolina flour

    2 tablespoons salt

    4 eggs (or substitute 2 cups chopped cooked nettles)

    Water, as needed

FOR THE FILLING

    2 cups finely chopped fresh nettles (or substitute spinach or cooked mushrooms)

    2 cups fresh whole milk ricotta cheese

    1 cup grated Parmesan cheese

    Salt and ground black pepper, to taste

To make the pasta, combine the flour and salt on a work surface and shape into a mound with your hands. Make a large well in the center and crack the eggs into it (or add the cooked nettles, if using). Use the tips of your fingers to mix the flour into the eggs, a little at a time, until combined. Knead until it forms a smooth dough, sprinkling with a little water as needed. With a rolling pin, roll out the dough on a flat floured work surface and cut into 1-inch strips. Keeping the rest of the dough damp under a wet tea towel, run each strip through a pasta machine to a thickness of about ⅛ inch.

Sprinkle a baking sheet with flour. Bring a large pot of salted water to boil.

To make the filling, stir together all the ingredients in a medium bowl. Using a small teaspoon, spoon dollops of filling onto a strip of rolled ravioli dough, about 2 inches apart. Carefully lower another strip on top. Press down firmly with a finger between the dollops, and slice the strips crosswise between the dollops to create rectangles. Using a fork, press all four edges of each ravioli, and space them apart in a single layer on the prepared baking sheet. Repeat with the remaining strips of dough and filling.

When the water is boiling, carefully drop about 10 ravioli into the water, one at a time. Cook until all the ravioli are floating and the edges are al dente, 3 to 5 minutes. Use a slotted spoon to lift them from the pot and place in a medium bowl. Drizzle with a little olive oil so they don't stick to each other, and repeat the process until all the ravioli are cooked. Spoon over them whatever sauce you choose.

Maitake Pizzetta by Constance Green

 immune support | MAKES 2 PIZZETTAS, OR ABOUT 4 SERVINGS

Constance Green, co-author of the *Wild Table* cookbook, shares this delectable recipe for using wild or cultivated maitake mushrooms. "Very few foods have the legendary immune-enhancing properties of maitakes," says Connie. "This marvelous quality, combined with its extraordinarily delicious flavor, makes maitake a magical food indeed." She says not only do maitakes grow abundantly in the wild, east of the Mississippi, but now they are also widely available as an organically cultivated mushroom.

Use a pizza dough of your choice, or make this into great crostini by toasting slices of sourdough bread and topping with this blend.

- 1½ to 2 pounds of maitake mushrooms (wild or cultivated)
- ¼ cup plus 2 tablespoons olive oil
- 1½ tablespoons finely chopped garlic
- 1 teaspoon sea salt, plus a pinch
- ¼ teaspoon ground black pepper
- 1 ball of pizza dough, or several 1-inch-thick slices of sourdough bread
- ¾ cup grated Parmesan cheese
- ¼ cup chopped fresh parsley

Heat the oven to 450°F. If the maitake are wild, clean them by brushing and rinsing them. Tear the maitake into loose petals (the more surface area you expose, the crispier they will get). Place them in a large bowl and add 3 tablespoons of the olive oil and the garlic, 1 teaspoon of the salt, and the pepper. Toss well. Spread out the mushroom mixture in a thin layer on a large baking sheet. Roast in the oven for 5 to 7 minutes, until the mushrooms are browned and fairly crispy.

Raise the oven temperature to 500°F to 550°F. On a floured work surface, roll out your pizza dough into thin, 6- to 10-inch circles. If using bread instead, toast lightly in the oven. (Watch it carefully so it doesn't get too toasted, because it will be going back into the oven again.)

Paint the surface of the pizza dough with the remaining 3 tablespoons of oil, leaving ½ inch around the edge without oil. If using bread, paint the entire surface of the toast with oil. Sprinkle a single layer of mushroom mixture over the surface and top with the Parmesan: 2 to 3 tablespoons on a pizzetta or 1 tablespoon on a large slice of bread.

Slide the pizzettas directly onto the hot oven rack. Bake for 8 to 10 minutes (the crostini for 4 to 5 minutes). Remove from the oven and place on a wire rack. Sprinkle with the chopped parsley and a pinch of sea salt.

Immune-Boosting Amaranth-Veggie Sauté or Salad by Zoe Petricone

➕ *immune support* | MAKES 4 TO 6 SERVINGS

Zoe served this grain and vegetable salad during one of my herbal school intensives, and it was a huge hit. We all loved this filling and delicious salad, with its depth of flavors and its bright citrus and herbal notes, and I noticed many people going back for seconds. The Brussels sprouts and cauliflower are rich in antioxidants and choline, the mushrooms are high in zinc, and the parsley is chock-full of vitamins and folic acid. Together with immune-supporting sage, thyme, and garlic, this healthy lunch or entrée makes a highly nutritious meal. To make this dish gluten-free, substitute brown rice or buckwheat for the barley. Serve hot, without the Parsley Dressing, or add the dressing, refrigerate, and serve chilled.

FOR THE SALAD

½ cup uncooked amaranth

½ cup uncooked pearl barley

1 cup uncooked quinoa

4 cups broth (see Broths and Stocks, page 192)

3 tablespoons extra-virgin olive oil or ghee

4 garlic cloves, minced

1 large onion, chopped

8 to 10 small Brussels sprouts, sliced in half

4 carrots, shredded

½ cauliflower, trimmed and chopped

Juice and zest of 1 lemon

8 to 10 crimini mushrooms, sliced

2 tablespoons balsamic vinegar

1 teaspoon chopped fresh sage

1 teaspoon chopped fresh thyme

1 teaspoon chopped fresh rosemary

1 teaspoon chopped fresh marjoram

Pinch of cayenne

Salt and ground black pepper, to taste

1 cup cooked chickpeas (if serving as a cold salad)

1 cup cherry tomatoes, sliced in half (if serving as a cold salad)

½ cup chopped red bell pepper (if serving as a cold salad)

FOR THE PARSLEY DRESSING

½ cup olive oil or Lemony Salad Oil (page 38)

¾ cup balsamic vinegar or Grape Leaf Vinegar (page 32) or Vinegar of the Four Thieves (page 33)

2 garlic cloves, minced

2 teaspoons minced fresh parsley

1 teaspoon prepared mustard

1 teaspoon honey or Nutritious Nettle Honey (page 54)

Salt and ground black pepper, to taste

Stir together the amaranth, barley, and quinoa in a medium saucepan. Pour in the broth, stir, cover, and bring to a boil over high heat. Reduce the heat to low and simmer for 15 minutes. Remove from the heat and set aside.

Heat the olive oil in a skillet over medium heat, add the garlic and onion, and sauté, stirring frequently, until the onions are translucent, about 5 minutes. Add the Brussels sprouts, carrots, and cauliflower and sauté for another 7 minutes. Stir in the lemon juice and zest. Add the mushrooms, balsamic vinegar, sage, thyme, rosemary, marjoram, cayenne, and a pinch of salt and black pepper, and cook, stirring often, for an additional 5 minutes. Adjust salt and pepper to taste.

To serve as a hot sauté, toss the cooked grains with the sautéed vegetables to mix well, and enjoy.

To serve as a cold salad, scrape the sauté into a bowl and cover the bowl with plastic wrap or a towel and refrigerate at least 2 hours. Remove the wrap and stir in the chickpeas, tomatoes, and bell pepper. To make the salad dressing, blend all the dressing ingredients together, then pour the dressing over the chilled salad and stir well. Serve chilled.

14

SWEET TREATS

THESE LOVELY DELICACIES are sweet ways to use medicinal and healing herbs. Herbs such as rose petals, violets, and even ginger, fennel, astragalus, and mineral-rich nettles have much to offer when paired with honey or sugar. Part of the magic of cooking with herbs is that their color and aromas shine through—and this is especially true when making these ice pops, shortbreads, puddings, jellies, jams, and candied seeds and flowers. Enjoy these sweet treats on special occasions and in moderation; some are wonderful for hot summer days and others are the perfect comfort food on cold wintry nights. Either way, be creative and let the whole family help harvest, prepare, and enjoy.

Immune Boost Ice Pop by Jan Berry

 immune support | YIELDS ABOUT 4 ICE POPS

It's easy and fun to take the idea of a tea or infusion one step further and turn it into an ice pop. The herbalist and *Nerdy Farm Wife* blogger Jan

Berry likes to gives this special, immune-boosting treat to her children when they're feeling under the weather.

- 1 handful of lemon balm leaves
- 3-inch piece of dried astragalus root
- 1-inch piece of fresh gingerroot, chopped
- 2 cups apple juice or water

Combine all the ingredients in a small saucepan over high heat. Bring to a boil, then reduce the heat to low, cover, and simmer about 15 minutes. Remove the pan from the heat and let it sit, covered, until it cools to room temperature. Strain into a liquid cup measure and pour into ice-pop molds. Freeze for several hours until solid.

Sweet Love Ginger Shortbread by Kirstin Uhrenholdt

 heart support | YIELDS ABOUT 40 COOKIES

My friend, private chef and author Kirstin Uhrenholdt, is well known for her delicious artistry in the kitchen. Here she shares a cookie that she says is "rich in contrasts . . . chewy, tender, sweet, and spicy. Plenty of candied ginger is the secret here, so stop by the bulk bins of your health food store." Ginger is a wonderful digestive aid, enlivening the digestive system and helping to ease bloating, gas, and indigestion. It is also traditionally used to stimulate the cardiovascular system and is a wonderful warming herb for the winter. "Brew a pot of tea," says Kirstin, "and get ready for your family and friends to be drawn to your kitchen table when you bake these mouth-watering cookies."

For quick sweets on busy days, Kirstin says to double or triple the recipe and freeze the cookie dough roll, to be cut and baked whenever you need it. Wrap aluminum foil around the parchment paper and label the roll with the baking directions. Store your treasure in the freezer, where it will last for at least 3 months.

- 1 cup (2 sticks) butter, at room temperature
- ½ cup firmly packed light brown sugar or coconut palm sugar
- 2 cups all-purpose flour
- 1½ cups roughly chopped candied ginger (pea-size pieces)
- ¼ teaspoon salt

In a large bowl, beat together the butter and brown sugar using a wooden spoon and vigorous arm movements. Continue to beat until the mixture is somewhat light and fluffy, then fold in the flour, candied ginger, and salt.

Rip off a few large pieces of parchment or wax paper and place on your work surface, with the short edge in front of you. Along the bottom of the short edge put a "roll" of cookie dough (you can use an ice cream scoop to do this, placing several 2-inch balls in a row). Tightly roll up the paper so that the balls smoosh together, leaving you with a long roll of cookie dough 2 to 3 inches in diameter. Repeat with the remaining dough. Chill the dough for at least 1 hour in the freezer.

Preheat the oven to 300°F. Grease 2 baking sheets. Take out the rolls, unwrap the dough, and cut them into thin slices. Arrange the cookies 1 inch apart on the prepared baking sheets and bake them until they are pale golden, 25 to 30 minutes. Transfer to a rack to cool completely. Store cooled cookies in an airtight container on the countertop for up to 5 days.

Nettle Rice Pudding

 calming | MAKES SIX TO EIGHT ½-CUP SERVINGS

I've always loved rice pudding, but I had never tried making my own until I was inspired to make herbal rice pudding, which seemed like fun. As it turns out, it was! This rice pudding is easy and fragrant and rather forgiving—all you need is extra hot tea or water on hand to adjust the texture. Begin your pudding with herbal tea instead of milk—it makes all the difference.

I originally attempted to make nettle pudding by steeping fresh nettle leaves in milk and then cooking raw rice in the strained milk. It didn't work: the milk burned, the rice didn't cook thoroughly, and the nettle flavor didn't come through. I experimented until I found this method, and the secret seems to be starting the rice in a liquid other than milk. In this recipe, the liquid is nettle tea. I also use nettle tea to thin the pudding as it cooks, which gives it a great creaminess. This recipe creates a luscious, lightly sweet, and very creamy pudding with a hint of nettle about it. It's very simple and quick to make. Whip it together to soothe tired bodies after a cold day out in the snow.

1½ cups Basic Nettle Infusion (see page 95)
1 to 1¼ cups uncooked Arborio rice
Pinch of salt

1 teaspoon butter

2 cups fresh (preferably raw) cow's milk or alternative milk of choice

¼ teaspoon ground cinnamon

¼ cup sugar

1 teaspoon vanilla extract

First, make the nettle infusion, using either fresh or dried nettle leaves. Strain and reserve the tea.

In a small heavy-bottomed saucepan, combine 1 cup of the nettle tea with the rice, salt, and butter over high heat. Bring to a light boil, then reduce the heat to low and simmer, stirring frequently until the rice is mostly cooked, about 20 minutes. Add more tea if necessary.

In medium heavy-bottomed saucepan, combine the milk, cinnamon, and sugar and place over medium-low heat. Heat to just below a boil, stirring frequently, then reduce the heat, and simmer for 5 minutes. Add the rice mixture to the milk mixture and increase the heat to medium. Cook, stirring frequently, until the rice is cooked and the desired consistency is reached, 5 to 10 minutes. Add the remaining ½ cup of nettle tea by the tablespoon to achieve the desired consistency, and taste the rice to make sure it is thoroughly cooked. Stir in the vanilla extract and serve immediately.

NOTE: The pudding will thicken as it sits, even in the refrigerator. If it does, add more hot tea, hot milk, or hot water to thin it, if desired.

Rose Petal Rice Pudding

 stress support | MAKES SIX TO EIGHT ½-CUP SERVINGS

In addition to being the symbolic flower of love, roses are often used to ease feelings of anger. Gypsy herbalist Juliette de Bairacli Levy suggests giving angry and exhausted children milk to soothe their emotional state. I think combining milk with rose petals is a lovely soothing remedy for anger, irritation, and frustration of any sort. This pudding is light, deliciously creamy, and quite fragrant. For an extra special treat, stir in some Rose Petal Jelly (page 223).

1 tablespoon shredded fresh rose petals, or 1 teaspoon crumbled dried

½ cup hot water

1 cup cold water

1 to 1¼ cups uncooked Arborio rice

Pinch of salt

½ tablespoon butter

2 cups fresh (preferably raw) cow's milk or alternative milk of choice

2 tablespoons dried rose petals (in tea strainers)

Two 2-inch cinnamon sticks

¼ cup sugar

1 teaspoon vanilla extract

1 to 2 teaspoons Rose Petal Jelly (page 223) or Rose Hip
    and Cranberry Jam (page 224), optional

First, make rose petal tea: Place the fresh rose petals in a very small bowl and cover with the hot water. Set aside.

In a medium heavy-bottomed saucepan, combine the cold water, rice, salt, and butter and place over high heat. Bring to a light boil, then reduce the heat to low and simmer, stirring frequently, until the rice is mostly cooked, about 20 minutes. Add more water if necessary.

In another medium heavy-bottomed saucepan, combine the milk, dried rose petals, cinnamon, and sugar and place over medium-low heat. Heat to just below a boil, stirring frequently, then reduce the heat, and simmer for 5 minutes. Add the rice mixture to the milk mixture and increase the heat to medium. Strain the rose petal tea into the pot. Cook, stirring frequently, until the rice is cooked and the desired consistency is reached, 5 to 10 minutes. Stir in vanilla extract and remove the cinnamon sticks. Stir in the jelly or jam, if using.

ROSE PETALS

Rosa spp., especially *Rosa rugosa*

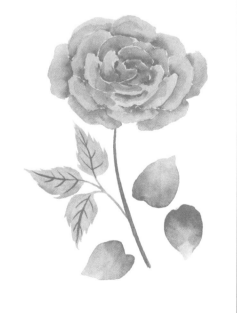

Versatile, subtle, and pleasing to the senses, roses have an ancient connection with people and have been used for centuries both internally and externally. Traditionally, rose petals have been used as nervine tonics to ease depression, anxiety, premenstrual syndrome (PMS), and grief. Many herbalists today prize roses for supporting the heart, both physical and emotional, and also for helping ease PMS symptoms and uterine congestion. Rose petals are delicious in teas, infusions, syrups, and especially in honeys; also use them in herbal milks and puddings alongside ashwagandha and holy basil (tulsi).

Rose Petal Jelly by Linda Lee Alley

Summer's bounty in a clear glass jar—what could be more appealing? Preserve the fresh scent of summer roses with this lovely canned jelly from Martha's Vineyard condiment crafter Linda Alley, who is well-known for her thirty original jams, jellies, and mustards. Linda says,

> My first sensual awareness of the *Rosa rugosa* plant was back in the mid-1970s, while sun bathing at Long Point Beach on Martha's Vineyard. The aroma wafting across the little pond behind the dune was intoxicating. I set about to find the source. It was all the beautiful, vibrant pink rose petals of the wild *Rosa rugosa* plants that grow all along the pond. It was mystical and heady. Picking fresh petals and then making an infusion is an experience for the senses.

Make this jelly with fresh rose petals and stir it into Rose Petal Rice Pudding (page 221). Alternatively, spread it on biscuits or tea cake, toast, or rice cakes; drizzle it on ice cream; include it in chutney recipes; or mix it into smoothies.

6 cups fresh, unsprayed *Rosa rugosa* petals (preferably pink), rinsed in a colander

7 cups sugar

1 tablespoon lemon juice

20 fresh rose petals, for garnish, optional

2 pouches liquid pectin

½ tablespoon unsalted butter, optional

Eight to ten ½-pint glass canning jars with lids

Put the 6 cups of petals in a large saucepan and add enough water to cover. Place over high heat and bring to a boil. The water will begin to turn bright pink. Reduce the heat to low and simmer for 20 minutes, stirring frequently.

Strain the infusion through a colander into a large bowl. Measure 4 cups of this infusion into a medium pot and set the rest aside for another use. Add the sugar and lemon juice to the pot and place it over high heat. Bring to a rolling boil, stirring constantly. Stir in the 20 rose petals, if desired, then add the pectin and stir well. Allow to come to a boil again and cook for 1 to 2 minutes. Remove from the stove. Add the butter, if desired, to rid the jelly of foam.

Prepare a water bath canner: fill with about 6 inches of water, place the canner rack on top, and bring to a boil. Prepare the canning jars and their lids by immersing them in a pot of boiling water or running them through a dishwasher. When the jelly mixture is ready, empty the jars and fill to within ¼ inch of the top with the hot jelly. (But don't let all the petals go into the first couple of jars!) Clean the rims with a moistened paper towel and screw on the lids. Carefully place each jar in the canner's rack and then lower the rack, ensuring the jars are covered by 1 to 2 inches of water. Boil for 7 minutes. Use a jar lifter to remove the jars from the canner and let cool on the countertop on a towel. Linda suggests turning the jars over several times while they are cooling to distribute the petals uniformly throughout the jar. Check the seals: the lids should be sucked down within about 10 minutes. The jam will last 3 to 4 weeks in the refrigerator once the jar is opened.

Rose Hip and Cranberry Jam by Kate Gilday

 immune support | YIELDS EIGHT TO TEN ½-PINT JARS

"Each fall our family would vacation on Cape Cod and enjoy gathering the abundant cranberries we found in the hidden bogs in the dunes," says the herbalist Kate Gilday.

We would wander with our baskets and discover these "rubies in the sand," gathering them for jam, sauce, breads, chutneys, and other tart delights. At the same time, we would keep our eyes open for the bright red, plump rose hips gracing the *Rosa rugosa* shrubs along the edge of the ocean sands. Once we moved to the Adirondacks, we found many hidden bogs filled with wild cranberries. We gather these plump, red berries from our canoes, or step carefully into the cool bogs. We also started growing *Rosa rugosa* shrubs in our yard and after several years began having a good-size crop of fat, delicious rose hips.

Preparing a jam or syrup from these two beautiful fruits is a wonderful way to celebrate the autumn bounty. Come winter, the bright warm color and sweet-tart taste remind us of the richness of life, the bounty of wild foods, and the adventures in discovering where they live.

Kate notes that you can also add hawthorn berries to this recipe, since they are another red berry ripe at this time of year. She adds that hawthorn berries have a bit of pectin in them that helps the jam to thicken. Enjoy this jam spread on biscuits or Wheat and Wild Seed Peasant Bread (page 173).

8 cups rose hips (harvested after the first frost)

3 cups cranberries

1 cup hawthorn berries, optional

2 teaspoons calcium water (made with the calcium packet included in commercial pectin packages such as Pomona's Universal Pectin)

2 tablespoons lemon juice

1¼ to 2 cups sugar

2 teaspoons pectin powder

Eight to ten ½-pint glass canning jars with lids

Wash the rose hips and remove the stems and black tips. (Removing the seeds helps avoid any bitter flavor but is optional.) Place in a medium heavy-bottomed pot with a small amount of water. Add the cranberries and the hawthorn berries, if using. Place over very low heat and cook until the cranberries are soft. Let cool.

Once cool, puree the fruit in a food mill set over a medium bowl. Use the back of a knife to scrape the puree from the outside of the mill into the bowl. Clean your pot. Measure 4 cups of the milled fruit into the clean pot and set the rest aside for another use. Add the calcium water and lemon juice and mix well with a spoon. Bring the fruit mixture to a full boil over medium-high heat.

In a small bowl, whisk the sugar and pectin powder well. Stir the pectin-sugar mixture into the hot fruit mixture and cook, stirring vigorously, until the pectin has dissolved and the jam has returned to a boil, 1 to 2 minutes. Once the jam is fully boiling, remove the pot from the heat.

Prepare a water bath canner: fill with about 6 inches of water, place the canner rack on top, and bring to a boil. Prepare the canning jars and their lids by immersing them in a pot of boiling water or running them through a dishwasher. When the jam mixture is ready, empty the jars and fill to within ¼ inch of the top with the hot jam. Clean the rims with a moistened paper towel and screw on the lids. Carefully place each jar in the canner's rack and then lower the rack, ensuring the jars are covered by 1 to 2 inches of water. Boil for 7 minutes. Use a jar lifter to remove the jars from the canner and let cool on the countertop on a towel. Check the seals: the lids should be sucked down within about 10 minutes. The jam will last 3 to 4 weeks in the refrigerator once the jar is opened.

HAWTHORN

Crataegus spp., especially *Crataegus monogyna*

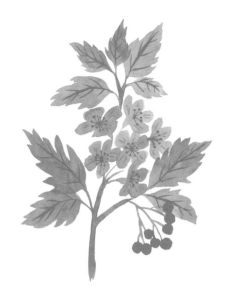

Prized as a cardiac tonic and for supporting the whole circulatory system, hawthorn's tart berries are taken in the form of a tea, tincture, paste, or even jelly to counter high blood pressure and arteriosclerosis. The Cherokee herbalist David Winston says the berries, leaves, and flowers of hawthorn (especially *Crataegus monogyna*) are useful for weakened heart muscle, venous integrity, and preventing deposits of plaque on arterial walls. Hawthorn is a gentle heart tonic, and is also astringent and useful against diarrhea. Hawthorn leaves and fresh and dried flowers have a lovely, pleasant, almost fruity taste and make a wonderful tea or infusion; also use them in syrups and honeys, and powdered (with their berries) in electuaries and smoothie blends. Fresh hawthorn berries can be made into jams.

VIOLET

Viola spp., especially *Viola odorata*

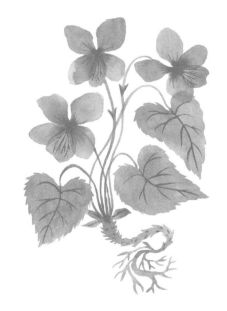

Colorful and sweet tasting, violet has long been used as a delicious food and a cooling, expectorant medicine. The leaves soothe bronchial congestion and irritation during both wet and dry coughs, and are traditionally used to help with indigestion. Applied topically, a wash, liniment, salve, or compress of the leaf and/or flower is not only soothing but also mildly styptic. Many successful first-aid ointments include violet leaf and flower, which are cooling and anti-inflammatory. Munch on the raw flowers, nibble raw leaves, and include the young, small leaves in salads; infuse both leaf and flower in vinegar or olive oil; and use violet in pestos, rice and grain dishes, sautés and stir-fries, salads, honeys, and elixirs.

Fruit Salad with Candied Violet Flowers

by Kate Gilday

 refreshing | MAKES 4 TO 6 SERVINGS OF FRUIT SALAD,
WITH 1½ CUPS CANDIED FLOWERS

This is a beautiful fruit salad that is quick to put together and deliciously sweet without added sugar. These fruits are high in antioxidants, plant chemicals that help maintain cell health in the body. Choose fruits that are in season where you live for the freshest taste. Top it with Kate Gilday's delicate candied violets to make this for a special occasion—or just to celebrate springtime! "We use the purple violets, and also the heartsease pansy for these candied flowers," says Kate. "My children loved making them when they were small, and then they were surprised when I served a birthday cake or some fruit with the pretty flowers decorating the special dessert. Or even better—they got to do it themselves!"

FOR THE FRUIT SALAD

3 cups nontropical fruits or berries, such as blueberries, raspberries, blackberries, huckleberries, chopped apples, plum slices, and/or peach slices

2 cups tropical fruit, such as banana slices, starfruit slices, kiwi slices, pineapple chunks, and/or papaya chunks

2 tablespoons yogurt (such as Citrus Yogurt, page 154) or Triple Berry Oxymel (page 75)

Juice of ½ lemon or lime, to taste

FOR THE CANDIED VIOLET FLOWERS

2 handfuls of violet flowers (or substitute rose petals)

¼ cup sugar

1 egg white

To make the fruit salad, gently stir together the nontropical and tropical fruits and the yogurt or oxymel in a medium serving bowl. Drizzle the lemon juice over the top and stir gently to combine. Cover the bowl and refrigerate.

Gather the flowers in the morning when they are fresh, but after the dew has dried. Line a baking sheet with parchment or wax paper. Pour the sugar onto a small plate.

To make the candied violets, beat the egg white in a small bowl until just frothy. Holding a very small paintbrush in one hand and a flower in the other hand, dip the brush into the egg white and "paint" both sides of the flower.

Dip the painted violets into the sugar before the egg whites dry (or hold the flower in one hand and sprinkle sugar over it with the other hand). Place the flower on the parchment paper and repeat until all the flowers are finished. Set aside to dry.

Ladle the fruit salad into individual serving bowls and gently sprinkle the candied flowers on top. Serve immediately. Store any leftover flowers in a single layer in a closed container out of direct sunlight for up to 3 months for use on future special projects.

Coconut Candied Fennel Seeds by Blaire Edwards

 digestive support *refreshing* | YIELDS ABOUT ½ CUP

"Fennel is one of my favorite vegetables," says my wonderful former herbal student Blaire Edwards. "I try to include it in any roasted-veggie dish that I do. The seeds, too, are delicious and make a great digestive treat for after heavy meals (especially during the holidays). These seeds also look great in a glass jar on the table, and are a great way to introduce herbal medicine to your food-loving friends."

2 teaspoons coconut oil
½ cup whole fennel seeds
¼ cup honey or pure maple syrup

Place a piece of wax paper on your countertop. Heat the coconut oil in a small saucepan over medium heat until warm. Add the fennel seeds and stir until well coated with oil, then add the honey. Toast the mixture until it is slightly browned and aromatic, 5 to 7 minutes. Scrape the mixture onto the wax paper and spread out in a thin layer—the thinner the layer, the easier it will be to break into pieces. Allow to cool completely. Once cooled, break the candy into pieces and store in an airtight glass jar on the countertop or table. Eat a few seeds after a meal, and be sure to chew thoroughly.

ACKNOWLEDGMENTS

Herbal tradition is long and sweet. Recipes and ideas such as these could not happen without the generous sharing of information, thoughts, successes, and failures by the many women and men who have experimented with using these plants and with creating delicious and healing blends from them. Many thanks to those intrepid folks who experiment, taste, test, and throw caution to the wind in exploring Mother Earth and all she has to offer.

Many thanks, also, to my friends and family who have supported me in the production of this book. It entailed a lot of recipe making and testing. Special, warm thanks and gratitude go to Laurisa Rich and Lisa Benson for the hours of fun and friendship given during the creation and testing of these recipes and many others. Thanks to Mary Bellebuono for sharing many of her family recipes over the years.

I owe much gratitude to the contributors to this book, who generously shared their own expertise and recipes so that this would be a well-rounded collection full of ideas for using herbs in wildly versatile and creative ways. You've honored me with your support, and I am excited to share your work and vision with those looking to nourish themselves with herbal foods and drinks. My thanks go to Linda Lee Alley, Blaire Edwards, Jan Berry, Heather Thurber, Hank Shaw, Connie Green, Cathy Walthers, Kate Gilday, Doug Elliott, Corinna Wood, Robin Rose Bennett, Juliet Blankespoor, Sharon Egan, Manya Williams, Suzanna Stone, Brittany Nickerson, Kirstin Uhrenholdt, Laurisa Rich, Jan Buhrman, Zoe Petricone, and Rosalee de la Forêt.

And special thanks to the ladies who shared their inspiring hearth-and-home stories with me, which were colorful inspirations for the recipes that complete this book: Deb Cini, Ashley Parkinson, Sally Apy, Molly Purves, Dale Julier, Velma Atkins, Gail Tipton, and Nancy Weaver. As always, it's the stories that create the heritage, the memories that create the traditions. And thankfully for us, it's the herbs and trees and flowers that make our hearth-and-home stories—and our heritage and traditions—so meaningful.

REFERENCES AND
SUGGESTED READING

Atlas, Nava. *Vegetariana: A Rich Harvest of Wit, Lore, and Recipes.* Boston: Little Brown & Co., 1984. Revised edition, 1993.

A vegetable lover's classic.

Bellebuono, Holly. *The Authentic Herbal Healer: The Complete Guide to Herbal Formulary and Plant-Inspired Medicine for Every Body System.* Bloomington, IN: Balboa Press, 2012.

An introduction to more than 130 of the world's herbs and their indications and uses based on body system, with an emphasis on formulary and blending.

Bellebuono, Holly. *The Essential Herbal for Natural Health: How to Transform Easy-to-Find Herbs into Healing Remedies for the Whole Family.* Boston: Shambhala Publications, 2012.

My collection of recipes for medicines for internal and external use, with a focus on thirteen versatile herbs for the beginner.

Bennett, Robin Rose. *The Gift of Healing Herbs: Plant Medicines and Home Remedies for a Vibrantly Healthy Life.* Berkeley, CA: North Atlantic Books, 2014.

A spiritual and ceremonial approach to using herbs for food and medicine by one of America's loveliest herbalists.

David, Laurie, and Kirstin Uhrenholdt. *The Family Cooks: 100+ Recipes to Get Your Family Craving Food That's Simple, Tasty, and Incredibly Good for You.* New York: Rodale Books, 2014.

Delicious and fun recipes by my friend, chef Kirstin, in sisterly collaboration with Laurie; together they make a team that has produced two wonderful and user-friendly books about bringing the family together at the table.

Gail, Peter. *The Dandelion Celebration: A Guide to Unexpected Cuisine.* Cleveland, OH: Goosefoot Acres Press, 1990.

All about the magic and wonder (and nutrition) of dandelions.

Gibbons, Euell. *Stalking the Healthful Herbs.* New York: David McKay, 1966.

A classic in foraging and using wild foods, written with love, humility, creativity, and a bit of sassy honesty.

Gladstar, Rosemary. *Rosemary Gladstar's Family Herbal: A Guide to Living Life with Energy, Health, and Vitality.* North Adams, MA: Storey Books, 2001.

Useful, creative, and down-to-earth, Rosemary shares a treasure trove of recipes.

Hoffmann, David. *The Herbal Handbook*. Rochester, VT: Healing Arts Press, 1988.

Instruction in formulary and using herbs for medicine. Very informative.

Johnson, Cait. *Cooking like a Goddess: Bringing Seasonal Magic into the Kitchen*. Rochester, VT: Healing Arts Press, 1997.

Kitchen witchery at its finest, with delicious and lovingly created recipes.

Katz, Sandor Ellix. *Wild Fermentation: The Flavor, Nutrition, and Craft of Live-Culture Foods*. White River Junction, VT: Chelsea Green Publishing, 2003.

Helpful for making all sorts of fermented foods and drinks. Inspiring, with detailed instructions.

Levy, Juliette de Bairacli. *Herbal Handbook for Everyone*. London: Faber & Faber, 1966.

A landmark publication; I turn to this book again and again.

Shaw, Hank. *Hunt, Gather, Cook: Finding the Forgotten Feast*. New York: Rodale Books, 2011.

Gorgeous photos, inspiring recipes.

Walthers, Catherine. *Raising the Salad Bar: Beyond Leafy Greens— Inventive Salads with Beans, Whole Grains, Pasta, Chicken, and More*. New York: Lake Isle Press, 2007.

One of my favorite go-to cookbooks for healthy foods and imaginative salads.

Weed, Susun. *Healing Wise* (Wise Woman Herbal series). Woodstock, NY: Ash Tree Publishing, 1989.

A down-to-earth approach to using wildflowers and "weeds" for natural health.

Weil, Andrew, M.D., and Rosie Daley. *The Healthy Kitchen: Recipes for a Better Body, Life, and Spirit*. New York: Alfred A. Knopf, 2002. First paperback edition, December 2003.

A commonsense approach to making healthy foods, with some herbs included.

RESOURCES

FOR LEARNING ABOUT HERBS

To learn more about edible and medicinal herbs, as well as about the herbal heritage and how you can apply it in your own life, please see the following educational resources and schools that have been established by the talented contributors to this book:

The Bellebuono School of Herbal Medicine (BSHM)

This comprehensive school offers a variety of programs for beginning, intermediate, and advanced students to understand herbal formulary and the heritage and practice of herbal medicine. I run the programs to be inspiring, educational, and uplifting. The BSHM offers distance (online) and on-site programs for training and certification. Register for the distance program or the 2-Week Herbal Training Intensive on the beautiful island of Martha's Vineyard, or a relaxing women's herbal retreat in some of the world's most scenic destinations. Located on Martha's Vineyard with events internationally. www.hollybellebuono.com.

Owlcraft Healing Ways

Directed by Suzanna Stone, this school of herbal medicine offers clinical consultations, herbal apprenticeships, and day classes. Located in Virginia. www.owlcrafthealingways.com

The Chestnut School of Herbal Medicine

Directed by Juliet Blankespoor, this school offers classes on medicinal herb cultivation and more. Located in western North Carolina. www.chestnutherbs.com

Wisewoman Healing Ways

Directed by Robin Rose Bennett, this program provides training, apprenticeships, workshops, consultations, and more. Located in New Jersey. http://wisewomanhealingways.com

Thyme Herbal

Directed by Brittany Nickerson, this herbal medicine company offers "The Art of Home Herbalism" with online courses, workshops, and apprenticeships. www.thymeherbal.com/art-of-home-herbalism/

FOR PURCHASING HERBS

Many of these establishments are places where I have purchased bulk dried herbs and powders for years; others have been suggested to me by fellow herbalists as high-quality favorite suppliers. Remember when buying your herbs that bulk dried herbs (cut and sifted) and dried powders have a shelf life of approximately one year (though I've had them last much longer when kept in a cool, dark place). And of course the best resource for herbs is your own backyard! The next best resource is your local herbalist, farm, gardener, food co-op, or farm stand. If none of these is available, or if you want to purchase dried or powdered herbs, check out these vendors:

Vineyard Herbs Teas and Apothecary

My retail and wholesale site specializes in handcrafted herbal and black teas, salves, syrups, liniments, herb powders, salts, vinegar extracts, and herbal tinctures. www.vineyardherbs.com

Sandy Mush Herb Nursery

Specializing in traditional culinary and medicinal herbs and scented geraniums, this North Carolina nursery's catalog contains close to 1,600 varieties of plants, including wildflowers, natives, and other perennials. Find seeds, seedlings, and live plants. www.sandymushherbs.com

Zack Woods Herb Farm

A Vermont certified-organic herb farm selling dried herbs and live plants. They collaborate with other herbalists, farmers, and researchers to develop and share knowledge about the cultivation and preservation of medicinal plants. www.zackwoodsherbs.com

Great Cape Herbs

An apothecary and medicinal herb farm on Cape Cod, Massachusetts. http://greatcape.com

Flower Power Herbs and Roots, Inc.

A lively herbal store and workshop space in the East Village of New York City. www.flowerpower.net

Herbalist and Alchemist

David Winston's site for his original tinctures and extracts. www.herbalist-alchemist.com

Mountain Rose Herbs

A large retail mail-order establishment with a big selection of certified organic herbs. www.mountainroseherbs.com

Organic Creations

Online resource for soap, lotion, and crafting supplies, including bulk dried herbs. www.organic-creations.com

Local Harvest

A website devoted to connecting farmers with customers. Find farms, CSAs, herbalists, and vegetable and honey producers in your area, or anywhere. www.localharvest.org

For a Scoby

Cultures for Health www.culturesforhealth.com/obtaining-a-kombucha-scoby

RECIPE INDEX BY BENEFITS

INDEX

ABOUT THE CONTRIBUTORS

LINDA LEE ALLEY
Linda has been the owner of New Lane Sundries Jams and Jellies on Martha's Vineyard since 1987. She can be reached at linda@newlanesundries.com.

ROBIN ROSE BENNETT
Robin is "a writer, green witch, an herbalist, a wise woman … one who loves the earth and gives voice to the healing wild food and medicine plants which surround us, and a teacher of Wisewoman Healing Ways of herbal medicine and EarthSpirit teachings." She is the author of the books *The Gift of Healing Herbs: Plant Medicines and Home Remedies for a Vibrantly Healthy Life* and *Healing Magic: A Green Witch Guidebook to Conscious Living*. She teaches workshops and leads apprenticeships in New Jersey. Find her at www.robinrosebennett.com.

JAN BERRY
Herbalist, blogger, and farmer Jan Berry lives on a small hobby farm in the Blue Ridge mountains of Virginia with her husband, two children, and assorted collection of goats, ducks, chickens, bunnies, dogs, and one cat—aptly named Rascal. You can find her online at www.thenerdyfarmwife.com.

JULIET BLANKESPOOR
Juliet is the director and primary instructor at the Chestnut School of Herbal Medicine in Weaverville, North Carolina, where she teaches the traditional art of bioregional community herbalism. In addition, she cultivates a diverse herb garden and apothecary, and enjoys dreaming up herbal concoctions in her free time. Juliet also shares her plant obsession through her herbal articles and botanical photography on her blog, *Castanea*. She directs a distance-learning herbal program, and her first book, *Cultivating Medicinal Herbs*, is available on her website and from booksellers. Visit Juliet at www.chestnutherbs.com.

JAN BUHRMAN
Chef, instructor, and caterer Jan Buhrman leads international workshops and retreats based on healthy eating and cooking. She offers culinary experiences on Martha's Vineyard, in Costa Rica, and beyond, directs Kitchen Porch Catering, and co-leads Dieta Way to help people reinvent the way they experience life through food. Information about her retreats, blog, and experiences can be found at www.kitchenporch.com.

ROSALEE DE LA FORÊT

Rosalee is a clinical herbalist and herbal educator who is passionate about helping people explore the art of herbalism and natural health. She works with people all over the world to guide them in finding natural solutions to their chronic health problems. Rosalee frequently teaches about herbalism at conferences and through her work as education director at LearningHerbs .com. She is the author of many articles, e-books, and courses about natural health and herbalism, including her Taste of Herbs course and Herbal Cold Care course. To learn more, download a free e-book by Rosalee, *Top 3 Herbs for Your Health,* at www.herbalremediesadvice.org.

BLAIRE EDWARDS

Blaire is an herbalist with a passion for making herbal knowledge available and accessible to all. She gathers inspiration from many directions, including her ocean-side, Martha's Vineyard herbal apprenticeship with Holly Belle-buono, her clinical studies with David Winston, and, of course, from the plants themselves. When she isn't working in the organic food and beverage world, you can find Blaire blending custom formulas for her brand Mindful Medicinals, vending at local markets, or walking in the woods searching for edible mushrooms and medicinal plants. Find her at www.blaireedwards.com.

SHARON EGAN AND MANYA WILLIAMS

Sharon Egan and Manya Williams launched their bicoastal juice company, JuiceWell, in 2012. On similar paths in very different environments—Sharon in Sun Valley and Santa Barbara and Manya in New York City—they met, realized their shared vision and values, and took a leap of faith to partner and create a new brand together. JuiceWell quickly became a thriving and expanding business. With sustainable growth in mind, Sharon and Manya plan to continue developing great products for healthful living and delivering fantastic customer and community service and appreciation. Visit them at www.facebook.com/juicewell.

DOUG ELLIOTT

A resident of North Carolina, Doug is a naturalist, herbalist, storyteller, basket maker, philosopher, and harmonica wizard. He has authored five books and performs a lively collection of traditional tales and ancient legends, flavoring them with regional dialects, lively harmonica riffs, and facts stranger than fiction. He is a first-rate backwoods entertainer and has produced a number of award-winning recordings of stories and songs, as well as books. Visit him at www.dougelliott.com.

KATE GILDAY

Kate is an herbalist, flower essence practitioner, and teacher who is presently completing training as an Ayurvedic Lifestyle Consultant and working with Collaborative Healing, a group of practitioners in upstate New York who address health care through a unique integrative network, educating the community and combining conventional medicine with expert complementary care. She brings her love of wild places, song, and healing to the workshops she presents throughout the Northeast. Visit her online store, Woodland Essence, at http://woodlandessence.com.

CONSTANCE GREEN

Connie is the owner of Wine Forest in Napa, California, and is co-author with Sarah Scott of the beautiful cookbook *The Wild Table: Seasonal Foraged Food and Recipes*. At the forefront of the foraging movement, Connie Green is a renowned "huntress," wild-food gatherer, and edible mushroom expert, purveying her foraged delicacies to restaurants nationally. Find her at www.thewildtable.net and www.wineforest.com.

BRITTANY WOOD NICKERSON

A practicing herbalist, health educator, and cook, Brittany designs a wonderful herbal calendar and directs Thyme Herbal in Amherst, Massachusetts. She offers popular classes, workshops, and apprenticeships both on-site and online. Find more about Brittany at her website and blog, www.thymeherbal.com.

ZOE PETRICONE

Zoe lived in Brooklyn for ten years and trained as an aesthetician in New York City, devoted to healing the skin and the body. Her passion is cooking nutritious food that is full of textures and flavors, that not only nourishes the body but also tastes delicious.

LAURISA RICH

Raised on Alaska's south coast, Laurisa spent her early adulthood living and working on boats and islands. She settled on Martha's Vineyard in 2001, where she embraced the rooted life and the joys of serving her garden.

HANK SHAW

Author of *Hunt, Gather, Cook: Finding the Forgotten Feast*, proprietor of the award-winning website *Hunter Angler Gardener Cook* (www.honest-food.net), and food writer for multiple publications, Hank describes himself as a constant forager, angler, hunter, gardener, and fan of farmer's markets. His second book is titled *Duck, Duck, Goose.*

SUZANNA STONE

Suzanna directs Owlcraft Healing Ways, a school of herbal medicine in central Virginia offering clinical herbal consultations; day classes in the herbal healing arts, traditional foodways, and plant spirit medicine; and an all-outdoor nine-month herbal apprenticeship. Owlcraft Healing Ways works to enable and empower those who hear the call of the plants, striving to bring forth each individual's ability and skills as a healer, to bring the power of herbal medicine back to the people. Visit Suzanna at www.owlcrafthealingways.com.

HEATHER THURBER

Heather is a twenty-year traditionally trained herbalist, working closely with plant medicine since 1994. A Kripalu-certified Ayurveda bodywork practitioner, Heather offers treatment sessions in her holistic studio located at Breezy Pines Farm; she is also a Master Gardener specializing in medicinal plants, flowers, and vegetables. A registered herbalist and certified aromatherapist with a certificate of natural product manufacturing, Heather handcrafts a collection of award-winning medicines, oils, skin care remedies, and soaps. Learn more about Heather's businesses at www.ayurveda-mv.com and www.breezypinesfarm-mv.com.

KIRSTIN UHRENHOLDT

Kirstin grew up on a fruit farm in Denmark, pickin' 'n' prunin' and making pie. Then, by a stroke of luck, she ended up on a cargo ship to Greenland, doing more dishes than you can imagine. She escaped and became a beer wench in Appenzelle, Switzerland, where she says they speak a language no one understands. Eventually she landed in Los Angeles and, lo and behold, was kidnapped by some actors, some heavy rockers, and some kosher people. Presently she is living happily ever after. Check out her publications at http://thefamilydinnerbook.com.

CATHERINE WALTHERS

Cathy is a food writer, private chef, and culinary instructor, leading workshops from her headquarters on Martha's Vineyard. Cathy's delicious recipes can be found in her many helpful and popular books: *Raising the Salad Bar*, *Soups and Sides*, and *Kale, Glorious Kale*. Register to join one of her many fantastic cooking classes at www.catherinewalthers.com.

CORINNA WOOD

Corinna is the director of the Southeast Wise Women Herbal Conference, a popular gathering for over a thousand women every fall in the mountains of North Carolina. Corinna is also the co-founder and former director of Red Moon Herbs, and she teaches a weeklong Wise Woman Herbal Immersion program that empowers women to reconnect with their own wise woman through local plants, deep nourishment, and self-love. Find her at www.sewisewomen.com.

ABOUT THE AUTHOR

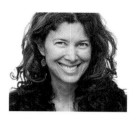

Award-winning traditional herbalist, empowerment speaker, and author Holly Bellebuono lectures at women's and business conferences, universities, and corporations, and leads retreats and workshops internationally about natural health; self-empowerment; symbolism and history; purpose, change, and transition; and herbal medicine. She is the author of several books, including *The Essential Herbal for Natural Health* and *Women Healers of the World*, winner of the 2015 Thomas DeBaggio Book of the Year Award by the International Herb Association. She has produced the audio CD collection *How to Use Herbs for Natural Health*, based on her book *The Authentic Herbal Healer*. This is Holly's fifth book.

Holly directs the Bellebuono School of Herbal Medicine, providing training and certification in herbal medicine. Her classes, hands-on workshops, retreats, and intensives enrich the student's understanding of natural health and the philosophy of healing, through both online and on-site seminars around the country.

A recognized formulator and herbalist, Holly founded Vineyard Herbs Teas and Apothecary, selling her original tea blends at Whole Foods Market, Stop and Shop, and other businesses in New England. She writes for a variety of publications, including *Taproot Magazine* and *SageWoman* magazine, and her work has been featured in *Parabola*, Britain's *Juno Magazine*, *Edible Vineyard*, *Mother Nature Network*, and more. She is a two-time Small Business Owner of the Year Award recipient and she leads goal-setting seminars for executive women and entrepreneurs.

Holly lives on Martha's Vineyard with her family.